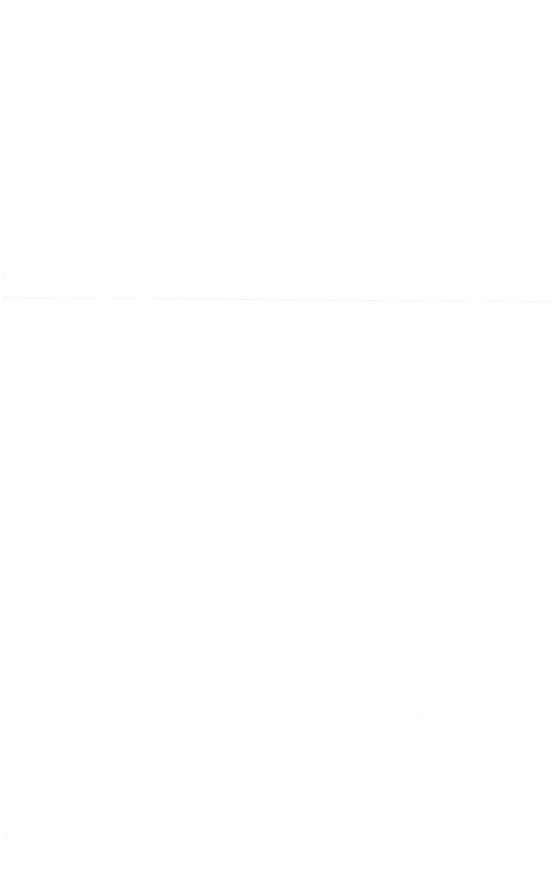

Pediatric Illnesses and Transition of Care

Guest Editor

VICKI L. ZEIGLER, PhD, RN

CRITICAL CARE NURSING CLINICS OF NORTH AMERICA

www.ccnursing.theclinics.com

Consulting Editor
JANET FOSTER, PhD, RN, CNS

June 2011 • Volume 23 • Number 2

SAUNDERS an imprint of ELSEVIER, Inc.

W.B. SAUNDERS COMPANY
A Division of Elsevier Inc.

Elsevier Inc., 1600 John F. Kennedy Blvd., Suite 1800, Philadelphia, PA 19103-2899

http://www.theclinics.com

CRITICAL CARE NURSING CLINICS OF NORTH AMERICA Volume 23, Number 2
June 2011 ISSN 0899-5885, ISBN-13: 978-1-4557-0433-0

Editor: Katie Hartner
Developmental Editor: Donald Mumford

Critical Care Nursing Clinics of North America (ISSN 0899-5885) is published quarterly by Elsevier Inc., 360 Park Avenue South, New York, NY 10010-1710. Months of issue are March, June, September, and December. Business and Editorial Offices: 1600 John F. Kennedy Blvd., Suite 1800, Philadelphia, PA 19103-2899. Periodicals postage paid at New York, NY and additional mailing offices. Subscription prices are $135.00 per year for US individuals, $282.00 per year for US institutions, $71.00 per year for US students and residents, $180.00 per year for Canadian individuals, $353.00 per year for Canadian institutions, $206.00 per year for international individuals, $353.00 per year for international institutions and $104.00 per year for Canadian and foreign students/residents. To receive student/resident rate, orders must be accompanied by name of affiliated institution, data of term, and the *signature* of program/residency coordinator on institution letterhead. Orders will be billed at individual rate until proof of status is received. Foreign air speed delivery is included in all *Clinics* subscription prices. All prices are subject to change without notice. **POSTMASTER:** Send address changes to *Critical Care Nursing Clinics of North America*, Elsevier Health Sciences Division, Subscription Customer Service, 3251 Riverport Lane, Maryland Heights, MO 63043. **Customer Service: 1-800-654-2452 (US and Canada); 314-447-8871 (outside US and Canada). Fax: 314-447-8029. E-mail: JournalsCustomerService-usa@elsevier.com (for print support) and Journals OnlineSupport-usa@elsevier.com (for online support).**

Reprints. For copies of 100 or more of articles in this publication, please contact the Commercial Reprints Department, Elsevier Inc., 360 Park Avenue South, New York, New York, 10010-1710; Tel.: (212) 633-3813, Fax: (212) 462-1935, and E-mail: reprints@elsevier.com.

Critical Care Nursing Clinics of North America is covered in *MEDLINE/PubMed (Index Medicus), International Nursing Index, Nursing Citation Index, Cumulative Index to Nursing and Allied Health Literature,* and *RNdex Top 100.*

Printed and bound by CPI Group (UK) Ltd, Croydon, CR0 4YY

Transferred to Digital Print 2011

Contributors

CONSULTING EDITOR

JANET FOSTER, PhD, CNS
Texas Woman's University, College of Nursing, Houston, Texas

GUEST EDITOR

VICKI L. ZEIGLER, PhD, RN
Assistant Professor, College of Nursing, Texas Woman's University, Denton, Texas

AUTHORS

VICTOR M. AQUINO, MD
Associate Professor of Pediatrics, Division of Pediatrics, Department of Pediatric Hematology/Oncology, University of Texas Southwestern Medical Center at Dallas, Dallas, Texas

LISA M. BASHORE, PhD, RN, CPNP, CPON
Nurse Practitioner and Program Manager of the Life After Cancer Program, Cook Children's Medical Center, Fort Worth, Texas

JISHA CHACKO, MS, RN
Family Nurse Practitioner, Lewisville, Texas

LYNN CLARK, MS, RN, BC, CPNP-PC
Nurse Practitioner and Manager, Pain Management Department, Children's Medical Center Dallas, Dallas, Texas

DOROTHY C. FOGLIA, RN, PhD, NEA-BC
Senior Director, Acute Care Services, Children's Medical Center, Dallas; Clinical Assistant Professor, College of Nursing, The University of Texas at Arlington, Arlington, Texas

PAUL C. GILLETTE, MD
Medical Director, Subspeciality Services, Denton, Cook Children's Healthcare System, Denton, Texas

CAROL J. HOWE, RN, MSN, CNS, CDE
Clinical Nurse Specialist, Diabetes Center for Children, The Children's Hospital of Philadelphia, Philadelphia, Pennsylvania

JULIE A. KOLINS, RN, BSN
Inpatient Clinical Nurse, Center for Cancer and Blood Disorders, Children's Medical Center, Dallas, Texas

KAY LAWRENCE, RN, MSN, CCRN, CPN
Senior Staff Nurse, Clinical Nurse Educator, Pediatric Intensive Care Unit, Medical
College of Georgia Children's Medical Center; Adjunct Faculty, Georgia Health Sciences
University College of Nursing, Augusta, Georgia

SUSAN MCCOLLOM, RN, ND, CPHON
Inpatient Clinical Manager, Center for Cancer and Blood Disorders, Children's Medical
Center, Dallas, Texas

LISA M. MILONOVICH, RN, MSN, PCCNP, CCRN
Pediatric Critical Care Nurse Practitioner, Team Leader, Advanced Practice Services,
Children's Medical Center, Dallas, Texas

PANTEA P. MINNOCK, RN, MSN, CRNP, CCRP
Pediatric Nurse Practitioner, Diabetes Center for Children, The Children's Hospital
of Philadelphia, Philadelphia, Pennsylvania

LINDY MOAKE, RN, MSN, PCCNP
Clinical Manager of Advance Practice Services, Heart Center, Children's Medical Center
of Dallas, Dallas, Texas

SAMUEL K. NDINJIAKAT, RCIS, MSPAS, PA-C
Pediatric Cardiac Catheterization Physician's Assistant, Heart Center, Children's Medical
Center of Dallas, Dallas, Texas

LINDA PAYNE, RN, BSN
Staff Nurse, Cardiac Intensive Care Unit, St Louis Children's Hospital, St Louis, Missouri

DONNA SALLEE, MS, RN, FNP-C
Minute Clinic, Fort Worth, Texas

BECKY SPENCER, MSN, RN
Graduate Research Assistant, College of Nursing, Texas Woman's University, Denton,
Texas; Doctoral Student, University of Kansas, School of Nursing, Kansas City, Kansas

CARA ZBYLUT, RN, BSN, CPON
Inpatient Clinical Nurse, Center for Cancer and Blood Disorders, Children's Medical
Center, Dallas, Texas

VICKI L. ZEIGLER, PhD, RN
Assistant Professor, College of Nursing, Texas Woman's University, Denton, Texas

Contents

Most healthy children receive more than 20 immunizations before 2 years of age. If the child is born with health concerns and is required to spend time in the neonatal intensive care unit, the number of painful encounters can reach into the hundreds. To optimally treat children with pain, nurses must realize that appropriately assessing and treating pain in children is a necessary part of their care.

The American Heart Association (AHA) has a strong commitment to implementing scientific research–based interventions for cardiopulmonary resuscitation and emergency cardiovascular care. This article presents the 2010 AHA major guideline changes to pediatric basic life support (BLS) and pediatric advanced life support (PALS) and the rationale for the changes. The following topics are covered in this article: (1) current understanding of cardiac arrest in the pediatric population, (2) major changes in pediatric BLS, and (3) major changes in PALS.

This article includes a definition of transition, the current state of transition, a review of transition research, an overview of chronic disease in survivors of childhood cancer (SCC), and the transition of SCC. In addition, models of transition are discussed, and the barriers to transition as well as principles for successful transition are identified.

Sepsis, septic shock, systemic inflammatory response syndrome, and Multiorgan dysfunction syndrome (MODS) remain clinical challenges in pediatric critical care. Understanding of the immune response has increased greatly over the past decade, which has certainly increased the understanding of the pathophysiology and treatment of these conditions. The future promises more exciting discoveries as we understand cellular physiology, immunity, and host responses even better. This article reviews the current knowledge about sepsis and MODS in pediatric patients and discusses the best treatment modalities while highlighting the critical aspects of nursing care for this vulnerable population.

Atrial septal defects (ASDs) have traditionally been repaired by surgical closure. Recently, transcatheter device closure has increasingly been used with excellent results. Comparative research evaluating long-term outcomes of transcatheter technique data reveal significantly fewer complications and shorter hospital stays than those reported for surgical repairs. This article reviews relevant literature comparing safety and efficacy, costs, and complications of transcatheter device procedures with surgical closure of ASDs.

Medical and nursing care of the hematopoietic stem cell transplantation (HSCT) recipient are complex because of the pathophysiology, HSCT process, pre-HSCT conditioning regimens, numerous medications and therapies, acute and chronic complications, adverse effects, resources involved, and environmental considerations. The HSCT process and therapies may affect any body system, requiring proficient and prioritized nursing care, possibly in an intensive care setting. Understanding the timing of potential adverse effects and complications based on engraftment will help provide competent, high-acuity care. Although autogenic and allogeneic HSCT are curative treatment options, there are numerous morbidity and/or mortality risks throughout the HSCT journey.

Pediatric critical care nurses are exposed to research in the critical care environment on a routine basis and should be knowledgeable about the ethical considerations inherent in this process. The following discussion includes information that centers on the ethical issues of conducting research with children. First, children as a vulnerable population is explored, followed by selected ethical principles that pertain to research, the role of the technological imperative in research, the process of informed consent, and finally, nursing considerations.

FORTHCOMING ISSUES

September 2011

Organ Transplant
Darlene Lovasik, RN, MN, CCRN, CNRN,
Guest Editor

December 2011

Cardiac Review
Bobbi Leeper, MN, RN, CNS, M-S, CCRN,
Guest Editor

March 2012

Pulmonary, Part I
Kathi Ellstrom, PhD, RN, ACNS-BC,
Guest Editor

June 2012

Pulmonary, Part II
Kathi Ellstrom, PhD, RN, ACNS-BC,
Guest Editor

RECENT ISSUES

March 2011

Sepsis
R. Phillip Dellinger, MD, MSc,
Guest Editor

December 2010

**Human Response to Disaster: Health
Promotion and Healing Following
Catastrophic Events**
Dana Bjarnason, PhD, RN,
Guest Editor

September 2010

Liver Failure
Dinesh Yogaratnam, PharmD, BCPS,
Sarah Saxer, PharmD, and
Tenita Foston, RN, MSN, FNP-C,
Guest Editors

THE CLINICS ARE NOW AVAILABLE ONLINE!

Access your subscription at:
www.theclinics.com

Preface

Critical care nursing of infants, children, and adolescents is different in many ways compared to the care of adults. Although great progress has been made in the diagnosis and management of acute and chronic health care conditions in pediatric patients, a myriad of challenges continue to exist. Children are not little adults; the physiology and subsequent pathophysiology of pediatric patients are constantly changing, requiring clinical skills that go beyond what nurses who care for adult patients are expected to have. Not only does the pediatric critical care nurse have a child to care for, there is also a family at the bedside that is an integral part of that child's care. The parents of these critically ill children are often stressed beyond their limits because of the suffering their child must endure, yet they are faced with making difficult decisions regarding their child's care. Pediatric critical care nurses are unique because their patients are unique; they must incorporate the parents of the patient into their plan of care and must deal with issues that seem incompatible with thoughts of a child, ie, pain, suffering, and sometimes death.

This issue of *Critical Care Nursing Clinics of North America* is a compilation of articles that provide information on a variety of topics related to illnesses seen in the pediatric population. One article discusses a unique aspect of caring for children with illnesses that occur in the pediatric age group, but that require care long into adulthood. The issue of transition of care is unique to the pediatric population owing to the fact that in the past, children with specific health care conditions such as cancer and congenital heart disease were not expected to survive to adulthood. Now, with better diagnostic techniques and state-of-the-art management strategies, these children are surviving well into adulthood, requiring that adult health care providers assume their care.

The first article, by Foglia and Milonovich, takes us back to the inception of pediatric critical care and pediatric critical care nursing. Along with this historical context, they provide an overview of the current state of the art of pediatric critical care nursing, including the role of technology, provision of a culture of quality and safety, establishing healthy work environments, and the roles of the patient and family as well as the nurse. Their article ends with a glimpse of how pediatric critical care nursing might look in the future. Next, Payne, Zeigler, and Gillette provide an overview of cardiac arrhythmias that occur in the immediate postoperative period following surgery for congenital heart disease. Mechanisms of these arrhythmias and diagnostic tools that can aid in their identification and management strategies are also reviewed.

In their article, Minnock and Howe discuss the role of continuous glucose monitoring systems in children with type I diabetes mellitus. They provide an overview of the products available for these children in addition to the benefits and barriers associated with their use. They also have included two case studies illustrating the use of these devices in the pediatric population. One of the constant issues that pediatric critical care nurses must address is that of pain and pain management in the children that they care for. Clark provides an excellent discussion of the definition and prevalence of pain in children, the child's physiologic responses to pain, barriers to optimal pain management in children, and achieving optimal pain relief in the acute care setting using pharmacologic and nonpharmacologic methods.

Crit Care Nurs Clin N Am 23 (2011) ix–x
doi:10.1016/j.ccell.2011.04.006
0899-5885/11/$ – see front matter © 2011 Elsevier Inc. All rights reserved.

The year 2010 resulted in the most notable change in the sequence of cardiopulmonary resuscitation in over a decade. Spencer, Chacko, and Sallee provide an overview of these changes, along with supporting rationale, with respect to pediatric basic and advanced life support. Bashore, in her article on the transition needs of survivors of childhood cancer, provides information on transition that is pertinent to many of the children in our care who will require transition to adult care as they near the end of adolescence. She includes models of transition, potential barriers to transition, and, finally, principles for successful transition.

One of the most challenging conditions that can occur in critically ill children is that of sepsis and multiorgan dysfunction syndrome. Lawrence describes the pathophysiology of each of these conditions and their effects on the various systems in the body, particularly how these conditions can be fatal in children if not properly managed. She includes the treatment of these disease entities in her discussion and provides information regarding the supportive role played by various bodily systems in that treatment. In their article, Moake and Ndinjiakat discuss the use of percutaneous catheters for the closure of atrial septal defects in children, one of the most common congenital cardiac defects seen in the pediatric population. They review traditional treatment options, but focus on the use of transcatheter closure with an emphasis on safety, efficacy, complications, and costs.

Kolins, Zbylut, McCollom, and Aquino provide a state-of-the-science article on the use of hematopoietic stem cell transplantation in children. This comprehensive review includes information regarding the types of hematopoietic stem cells, disorders that are amenable to this type of therapy, how these cells are collected, environmental considerations, and the actual process of hematopoietic stem cell transplantation, including before, during, and after transplantation. Their discussion continues with potential acute complications of the procedure, late effects of the procedure, and the specialized nursing care needed for these patients. My own article appears at the end of the issue and provides information pertinent to the ethical considerations associated with pediatric critical care research. Selected ethical principles, the technological imperative, the process of informed consent, assent, and parental permission as they apply to the research process and the role of the nurse are delineated.

Finally, as the guest editor of this issue of *Critical Care Nursing Clinics of North America*, I would like to thank each of the contributing authors for taking the time to provide their clinical expertise in this type of forum, a forum that will be used to disseminate this information worldwide. I would also like to thank Katie Hartner from Elsevier for her gentle reminders and enduring patience. The collective information provided here on Pediatric Illnesses and Transition of Care will undoubtedly be of benefit to pediatric critical care nurses across the illness spectrum and may even challenge some of them to alter how they provide their care. The rapidity at which technology is advancing and management is constantly changing requires that pediatric critical care nurses who care for children with acute and chronic health conditions remain at the forefront of knowledge acquisition in their fields.

Vicki L. Zeigler, PhD, RN
College of Nursing
Texas Woman's University
PO Box 425498
Denton, TX 76204, USA

E-mail addresses:
vzeigler@twu.edu; vickize@msn.com

The Evolution of Pediatric Critical Care Nursing: Past, Present, and Future

Dorothy C. Foglia, RN, PhD, NEA-BC[a,b,*],
Lisa M. Milonovich, RN, MSN, PCCNP, CCRN[c]

KEYWORDS

- Critical care nursing • Pediatric critical care nursing
- Children's hospitals • Pediatric intensive care units
- Medical/information technology • Healthy work environment
- Patient and family centered care

Children are different from adults and require health care that focuses on their unique needs. More importantly, children need extra time to act, extra monitoring, specialized medications, and atraumatic care. Pediatric nurses understand these distinctive needs of the patients and their families.[1] This extra care may not be captured by standardized patient acuity tools but may be better assessed within the context of the synergistic relationship between the competencies of the nurse and needs of the patients.[2] Caring for critically ill children in the pediatric intensive care unit (PICU) takes pediatric nursing to an entirely different and more demanding level. These nurses are specialists within a specialty.[3] PICU nurses, an almost forgotten subgroup of critical care nurses, face issues unique to caring for critically ill children and their families. On a daily basis, these nurses care for children who are in pain, who are suffering, and sometimes who are dying.[4] Pediatric critical care is a challenging arena for nurses. The children, families, and nurses form an interdependent triad in which the nurses' skill is vital in anticipating the needs of the patients and their family.[5]

Although current nursing literature is overflowing with information related to the history of nursing in general, and even pediatric nursing, very little is published about PICU nursing. The evolution of pediatric critical care nursing is presented based on

The authors have nothing to disclose.
^a Acute Care Services, Children's Medical Center, 1935 Medical District Drive, Dallas, TX 75235, USA
^b College of Nursing, The University of Texas at Arlington, Arlington, TX, USA
^c Advanced Practice Services, Children's Medical Center, 1935 Medical District Drive, Dallas, TX 75235, USA
* Corresponding author. Acute Care Services, Children's Medical Center, 1935 Medical District Drive, Dallas, TX 75235.
E-mail address: dorothy.foglia@childrens.com

Crit Care Nurs Clin N Am 23 (2011) 239–253
doi:10.1016/j.ccell.2011.02.003
0899-5885/11/$ – see front matter © 2011 Elsevier Inc. All rights reserved.

ccnursing.theclinics.com

a historical context, the current state, and future projections. More specifically, this treatise focuses on the environment, the patient and family, and of course, the PICU nurse. Concluding remarks provide an insight into how health care reforms and how the use of clinical information technology will affect the role of the pediatric critical care nurse in the future.

THE HISTORY OF CRITICAL CARE NURSING

The concept of critical care nursing has existed since Florence Nightingale wrote more than a century ago about the advantage of segregating hospital patients recovering from surgery. According to the Society of Critical Care Medicine (SCCM) mechanical ventilation of patients became possible, after World War II. The care and monitoring of these patients was more effective and efficient when they were grouped in a single location.[6] This quickly became the standard of care, and by the late 1950s, at least 25% of community hospitals with more than 300 beds had established intensive care units (ICUs).[6] Critical care medicine developed out of the needs of other subspecialties to provide care for the most critically ill patients. Advances in technology, further understanding of the pathophysiology of critical illness, and the development of multidisciplinary teams made this care possible. Specialization within the nursing profession followed suit, and modern critical care nursing emerged. The first special care unit for acutely ill patients opened in 1953 at North Carolina Memorial Hospital, Chapel Hill, North Carolina.[7] According to the SCCM, the first multidisciplinary ICU was created in 1958 at Baltimore City Hospitals, now Johns Hopkins Bayview.[8] This ICU led the way for optimal medical and nursing care to critically ill patients 24 hours a day and was also the first ICU covered by an in-house physician. Also, during the 1950s, an important finding relative to the evolving complexities of patient care in the ICU environment and nursing was exposed. Referenced as a triad, the necessities for safe ICU patient care included nursing expertise, the ability of the nurses to observe their patients, and adequate nurse staffing.[9]

Perhaps the most fascinating account of the history of critical care nursing is that of Jacqueline Zalumas.[10] Her research provided in-depth insight into the experiences of nurses from the emergence of critical care nursing in the 1960s through its evolution during the 1970s and 1980s. One interesting fact this research uncovered about the early development of critical care nursing was that these nurses took it upon themselves to learn how to use all the new technology in the ICUs. Zalumas[10] also found that the factors that nurses identified as most stressful about critical care were ironically the same ones they found to be rewarding. The most significant conclusion reached by this study is that the nurse became the most persistent treatment figure in the critical care unit because of skill, competence in judgment, and round-the-clock presence.

THE HISTORY OF PEDIATRIC CRITICAL CARE NURSING

As in the history of critical care nursing in general, some of the first references related to pediatric nursing also date back to the writings of Florence Nightingale. Her text, *Notes on Nursing*, was initially published around the time when the first children's hospital was opened in London.[11] Nightingale is oftentimes referred to as the mother of general nursing; however, what is less noted about her is that she was one of pediatric nursing's greatest treasures as well. Nightingale's love for children is everywhere in her writing. Her emphasis on children's nursing care needs is illustrated in this excerpt from *Notes on Nursing*, "It is a real test of a nurse whether she can nurse a sick infant."[12] Her concerns long ago about not having enough nurses to care for sick children, an occupation she viewed as particularly demanding, seem to be a trend nursing is experiencing today and quite possibly will continue in the future.

In the 1970s and 1980s, pediatric critical care nursing became more specialized with respect to the delivery of patient care. As available resources became more sophisticated, so did the preparation and requirements for working in the PICU. Nurses did not come to the PICU with these skills; it was common to have to educate nurses to the intricacies of the PICU.[5] A more detailed discussion of this evolution follows in a later section.

The role of nursing has been absolutely central to the evolution of PICUs (Levin DL, unpublished data, 2010). Fairman and Lynaugh[13] trace the evolution of critical care nursing from the battlefields and hospital recovery rooms of earlier decades to the contemporary units of today. They discuss the social, political, and economic factors that have led to the growth of critical care nursing.[13] This historical study reveals the importance of critical care in the US health care delivery system and the crucial role critical care nurses played in the shaping and delivery of this care. In the PICU, the nurse's influence continues.

FIRST CHILDREN'S HOSPITALS

Children's hospitals were highly visible in the communities where they were established. Medical and nursing staff who worked there prided themselves on providing a social safety net for all ill or abandoned infants and children who needed care. Children's hospitals also instilled energy for the promising specialties of pediatric nursing and medicine because of the opportunities for training, the feeling of shared identity and unity, and the research opportunities indigent hospitalized children provided.[12] According to the National Association of Children's Hospitals and Related Institutions (NACHRI), the origins of children's hospitals did not occur in the US.[14] In 1821, National Children's Hospital in Dublin was among the first hospitals in the English-speaking world devoted exclusively to the care and treatment of sick children. Dr Charles West, one of the hospital's founders and the one who had received medical training in Paris and Bonn where children's health care was far more advanced, moved to London 30 years later and helped launch the Great Ormond Street Hospital, which opened on February 14, 1852.[14] Soon after, Dr Francis W. Lewis of Philadelphia founded the first children's hospital in the US. The Children's Hospital of Philadelphia (CHOP) was opened in 1855, and the first US school of pediatric nursing was also launched at CHOP in 1895.[14] Today, there are more than 195 NACHRI member institutions, representing 80% of all children's hospitals. Of this number, approximately 50 are freestanding acute care children's hospitals and teaching hospitals.[14]

We would be remiss if we did not discuss our own roots here in Dallas, Texas, especially because it was a nurse who is truly recognized as the founder of Children's Medical Center (also known as Children's). Children's traces its beginning to the summer of 1913 when a group of nurses, led by the public health nurse May Forster Smith, organized an open-air clinic on the lawn of the old Parkland Hospital, fondly remembered by all as The Baby Camp.[15] What began from nurses recognizing that children received better care when focused only on them, grew into the Bradford Hospital for Babies, which joined the Children's Hospital of Texas and Richmond Freeman Memorial Clinic in 1947 as part of Children's. In 2008, Children's opened a second hospital at Legacy, Plano, to serve a greater number of patients in the area.

FIRST PICUS

Pediatric critical care medicine emerged in the 1960s, from its roots in general pediatric and cardiac surgery, adult respiratory care medicine, neonatology, and pediatric anesthesiology.[16] The first PICUs opened only after patient outcomes were realized when specialized care was provided to critically ill neonates and adults. Actually, the early PICU programs were not conducted in the US. These pioneers are from Sweden (1955, 1961), France (1963), Australia (1963), and London (1964).[7,17] In January 1967, Dr John J. Downes and his colleagues opened the first physician-directed multidisciplinary PICU at CHOP.[7,13] This first PICU was an outgrowth of a hospital-wide respiratory intensive care service and consisted of 6 fully monitored beds, with an adjacent procedure room and laboratory. Immediately after CHOP opened, other PICUs followed, such as at Children's Hospital of Pittsburgh and Yale-New Haven Medical Center in 1969 and Massachusetts General Hospital, Boston, in 1971.[17] The first PICU in Dallas was opened at Children's. Dr Theodore Votteler, Chief of Pediatric Surgery at Children's in 1975, recruited Drs Dan Levin and Frances Morriss to staff the PICU on a full-time basis.[13]

By the end of the 1970s, medical training programs developed for pediatric intensivists, and in 1985, the American Board of Pediatrics recognized Pediatric Critical Care Medicine as a specialty. Nursing programs followed suit, and by the mid-1980s, advanced practice/acute care nursing programs were established at Yale University, the University of Pennsylvania, and the University of California in San Francisco. Today, PICUs are found in every major medical center that provides care for critically ill pediatric patients around the world.

AMERICAN ASSOCIATION OF CRITICAL-CARE NURSES

A discussion of the evolution of critical care nursing would not be complete without a discussion about the relevance of a professional organization that has supported the role of the PICU nurse. As the largest specialty organization in the world, the American Association of Critical-Care Nurses (AACN) is dedicated to meeting the needs of critical care nurses who care for acutely and critically ill patients and their families. The AACN was first organized in 1969 as the American Association of Cardiovascular Nurses, and later in 1971, the association adopted its current name.[18] In 1982, the AACN responded to requests from members for specialized information, networking, and education by introducing Special Interest Groups (SIGs).[7] The pediatric SIG (under the leadership of Mary Fran Hazinski and colleagues) provided the first formal opportunity for PICU nurses to collectively assemble and share their expertise. Today, the AACN provides practice and educational and professional resources for approximately 500,000 critical care nurses with the vital responsibility of caring for critically ill patients. Building on decades of clinical excellence, the mission statement of AACN is to provide and inspire leadership to establish work and care environments that are respectful, healing, and humane.[19]

THE PRESENT

Today's contemporary critical care nurses are an essential aspect of the critical care team. Because critical care patients need continuous vigilance, critical care nurses contribute to improved patient outcomes and reduced patient morbidity and mortality, complications and errors, and overall costs.[20] Rapid advances in health care and technology have contributed to keeping more patients out of the hospital. However, patients in the PICU are more ill than ever and would not have survived in the past.[21] As patients become more medically complex, children's hospitals of today essentially have become one large critical care unit. Patients who were typically found in critical care units are now found in general units. Within the present environment, the triad (nursing expertise, the ability of the nurses to observe their patients, and adequate nurse staffing) previously discussed is even more important to contemporary nursing, in and out of the critical care setting.

The Environment

The role that the physical environment plays in the successful management of critically ill children must not be overlooked.[22] A well-designed PICU facilitates the work of the entire health care team, as well as supports the needs of privacy, comfort, and safety for the patient and family. It is vital for the PICU and room design to be adaptable and expandable while maximizing the resources of space, time, equipment, communication, and people. Although PICUs are designed within the confines of regulatory parameters, prioritization of space usually falls under 3 categories: patient care areas, support services, and family needs.

Today, most PICUs have only private rooms. Patient rooms are most often designed within 3 spacial concepts: patient, family, and staff. This shift is driven not only by safety, especially infection control practices, but also by the movement toward patient and family centered. PICUs have customized the space within the PICU patient room and the unit overall to accommodate the patient and the family.

Perhaps the most unique responsibilities of the PICU nurse hinge on being sensitive to the child's perceptions of the environment and the parents' fear and feelings of helplessness. Akin to this frame of reference is the realization that nurses are vulnerable too. It is not possible to deal with sick and dying children and not share some of the pain and grief.[5]

Medical and Information Technology

Hospitals are complex and oftentimes chaotic places.[23] In the PICU, this complexity is due in part to the critical nature of the patients' conditions. Today, however, the complexity also arises from the technologies that are not seamlessly connected to each other, including electronic health records (EHRs), biomedical devices, and robotic devices. According to a study by Hendrich and colleagues,[24] less than one-fifth of the nursing practice time was spent on direct patient care activities, such as providing procedures and treatments at the bedside, and only 7.2% of nursing time was spent on patient assessment and vital signs. Hendrich and colleagues assert that new practice models are needed that focus on the contributions of nurses by changing the way patient care is organized and delivered. The acute care setting (including the PICU) is being rapidly reshaped by medical and information technology. Hendrich and colleagues recommend that to transform care at the bedside in acute care, nurses must focus on 5 core concepts: leveraging the power of the EHR; achieving a balance among technologies, business models, and human needs; implementing rapid translation teams and interdisciplinary teams of designers; and creating an infrastructure for rapid network exchange of successful system design innovations.[24]

The Alliance for Nursing Informatics (ANI) purports that it is essential for nurses today and in the future to be engaged as leaders in the effective use of information technology to affect the quality of health care services.[25] Thus, nurses must be supported in an environment that enables their work as (1) leaders in the effective design and use of EHR systems; (2) integrators of information; (3) full partners in decision making; (4) care coordinators across disciplines; (5) experts to improve quality, safety, and efficiency and reduce health disparities; (6) advocates for engaging patients and families; (7) contributors to standardize the infrastructure within the EHR; (8) researchers for safe patient care; and (9) educators for preparing the workforce.[25]

Culture of Quality and Safety

Although patient safety is fundamental to patient care, the job of keeping patients safe has become more difficult. Critical care nurses work in chaotic practice environments, where patient acuity is high, patient and family needs are increasingly more complex, and human and fiscal resources are strained.[26] There is no question that nurses' vigilant surveillance, early detection, and timely interventions keep patients safe.

Critical care nurses are leading the way in defining medical and health care issues. In a national study conducted by VitalSmarts in partnership with AACN, it was reported that there are 7 crucial conversations that people in health care frequently fail to hold that likely contribute to avoidable errors and other chronic problems in health care.[27] The study found that these 7 categories of conversations are difficult yet at the same time, essential for all of those who work in health care settings to master. The most crucial concerns identified by the study participants included broken rules, mistakes, lack of support, incompetence, poor teamwork, disrespect, and micromanagement. It was concluded that it is critical for hospitals to create a culture of safety, where all members of the health care team can approach each other about their concerns.

More sophisticated, better, and increased use of technology has advanced the care of critically ill children.[13] These rapid changes, combined with an ever-changing state, have also created an environment with increasing errors and complications. This transformation necessitates a greater need for a humane and caring environment for patients and their families, as well as a requirement for all PICUs to establish and sustain a culture of quality and safety.

On July 9, 2008, The Joint Commission (TJC) released *Sentinel Alert 40* that outlined behaviors that undermine a culture of safety.[28] The alert is based on the single concept that working relationships between health care providers affect patient outcomes. PICU nurses do many things to improve their clinical knowledge and expertise, and it is highly believed that this is all necessary to ensure quality patient care. What continues to be a challenge is learning to be great communicators in a manner that strengthens trust and creates respectful relationships.[29] Healthy work environments discussed in the next section address this very mandate.

Healthy Work Environment

A stable infrastructure is required to achieve a healthy work environment. The AACN[30] has developed a program that can transform the environment in the PICU to one that supports a culture of retention. The link between healthy work environments, patient safety, and nurse retention is indisputable. An adequate supply of appropriately trained PICU nurses must be ensured, and those nurses who already work in the PICUs should also be retained. The AACN[31] recognizes the inextricable associations among the quality of the work environment, excellent nursing practice, and patient care outcomes. If PICU nurses are required to make optimal contributions to caring for patients and their families, establishing and then sustaining a healthy work environment is a priority.

The *AACN Standards for Establishing and Sustaining Healthy Work Environments* provide a solid infrastructure for this recommendation.[31] The 6 standards for establishing and sustaining healthy work environments represent evidence-based and relationship-centered principles of professional performance. The standards align with the core competencies for health care professionals outlined by the Institute of

Medicine (IOM), contribute to the implementation of elements in a healthy work environment articulated by the Nursing Organizations Alliance, and support the core competencies for nurse leaders identified by the Robert Wood Johnson Executive Nurse Fellows Program.[31] These standards include skilled communication, true collaboration, effective decision making, appropriate staffing, meaningful recognition, and authentic leadership. PICU leadership teams and nurses should use these standards as a foundation for thoughtful reflection and engaged dialogue about the current realities of the PICU work environment. Nurses are attracted to, are successful in, and stay in environments where they feel compensated, competent, and cared for.[32] It is important for nursing leadership to implement the interventions and transition to a healthy work environment that benefits the nurses and, ultimately, the patients and families.

The Patient and Family

The face of patients and families who seek critical care services has changed dramatically over the last few decades. In the past, many children with chronic or critical illnesses did not survive the disease that put them in the PICU. As medical knowledge and technology have advanced, so have the survival rates of children with congenital and acquired diseases. This increase has created a population of children with chronic comorbid conditions, not unlike adults, who are repeat recipients of critical care services. It is estimated, for example, that more than 800,000 patients with congenital heart disease have now survived to adulthood.[33] This same trend has been seen in patients with sickle cell disease, cystic fibrosis, childhood cancer, and other diseases. In addition, the number of technology-dependent patients who survive past infancy has also increased. For large children's hospitals, the prevalence is quite high, estimated at 20%, such that 1 in 5 children discharged from the hospital depends on technology in some way.[34] And more alarming is the fact that 1% of the technology-dependent children needed a ventilator.[34] Providing care for these patients requires the coordinated effort of many team members because their needs are often complex.

Twenty-five years ago, most ICUs were closed and only allowed family members to visit for short periods during the day; nowadays, the environment, both in physical design and staff attitudes, is much more open to families and encourages their participation in the care of their child. This change is particularly important given the new group of complex patients with long-term needs. Patients and family centered care is a concept that has been discussed in the literature since the 1970s; however, its actual movement into practice has taken years to institute and remains a work in progress in some organizations. Professional organizations such as the AACN, the Emergency Nurses Association, the American College of Critical Care Medicine (ACCM), and the American Academy of Pediatrics have released statements or standards of care surrounding family-centered care or family presence.[35–38] The releases include participation in the care of their child or family member as well as presence during rounds and/or during resuscitation and invasive procedures.

The ACCM Task Force has developed recommendations regarding visitation in PICUs and neonatal ICUs.[39] These include that (1) parents be permitted open visitation 24 hours a day, (2) siblings be allowed to visit with parental approval and after previsit education and (3) siblings of immunocompromised patients be allowed to visit with physician approval. These conditions have warranted modified layouts of the PICU to facilitate these activities and visitors and to provide sleeping spaces for parents, most often in the patient's room.

The movement of families out of the waiting rooms and to the child's bedside poses many additional challenges for the bedside nurse. A study by Aronson and colleagues[40] evaluated the effects of family presence on work rounds in PICU and its effects on family satisfaction, resident teaching, and the length of the rounds. They found that family presence during rounds provided high satisfaction but that families required significant attention on the first day of admission. Residents who participated in the study thought that their teaching was decreased as a result of family presence. Duran and colleagues[41] evaluated attitudes and beliefs about family presence. Their study revealed that clinicians had a positive attitude toward family presence but did express concern about safety, a family member's emotional response, and performance anxiety. This observation was less true of nurses than their physician colleagues. Petersen and colleagues[42] concluded from their evaluation of patient and family centered care practices among neonatal ICU and PICU nurses that although nurses agreed that the elements of patient and family centered care were necessary, they did not consistently apply them in daily practice. The investigators also noted that years of experience negatively affected these practices.

Parents obviously experience significant stress when their child is in the PICU. There are multiple studies in the literature that address causes of parental stress and nursing responses.[43,44] Most of these studies suggest that if the parents perceive the nurse as competent and caring, their stress is reduced. All these factors affect the current nurse's role at the bedside and provide the backdrop for nursing education and preparation in the future.

The Nurse

Nursing has also changed from that of 20 years ago. According to a US Department of Health and Human Services report, the average age of nurses in 2008 was 47 years, a significant increase from past decades.[45] This increase affects current practice at the bedside and will affect nursing in the future. Nurses entering the critical care arena come from multiple generations, which directly affects education, patient care, peer interactions, and retention. A growing number of nurses are entering the profession in their late 20s and early 30s because nursing is increasingly becoming a second career choice.[46]

In the early 1980s, most new graduates were required to complete an assigned period on a medical-surgical floor before entry into critical care; this is no longer the case. As a result of this influx of new graduates into critical care units, extensive orientation or internships have developed in most organizations. The goal of these programs is to integrate the knowledge gained by new graduate nurses in their academic education with that they will need to function in their new work environment. The programs are expensive for organizations, thus integration of multigenerational learning methods is important to the retention and financial feasibility of these programs. The literature suggests that there is a distinct difference in the views and values, because they relate to work and outside life, of baby boomers (1941–1964), Generation Xers (1965–1980), and Generation Y or Millennials (after 1980).[47–49] According to Wilson and colleagues,[49] those from the baby boomer generation report overall greater job satisfaction than those in the younger generations. This information directly affects the retention strategies used by employers and will likely lead to changes in these practices in the future.

In the opening session of the 15th annual Society of Pediatric Nurses conference, Dr Lynn Wieck challenged the conference participants to consider the depth of pediatric nursing. Her inspirational presentation highlighted the need to merge the strengths of the aging and knowledgeable nurse with those of the young and evolving nurse. Both of these generations at work will mutually benefit from each other and represent a powerful workforce in pediatric health care.[50] The PICU is not an exception to this challenge. As operating margins of hospitals shrink and expenses increase, a more creative workforce plan will be required. There will be less room for new graduate nurses and more reliance on more experienced staff to carry the burden of more complex care.

Before the early 1980s, literary and educational resources for nursing in pediatric critical care were scarce.[7] At present, several textbooks, both nursing specific and multidisciplinary, are available as a resource to nurses. Readily available access to the Internet and online databases, such as CINAHL and Ovid MEDLINE, has also opened up the available literature to the nurse at the bedside. In addition to written literature, professional organizations, such as the AACN and the SCCM, present conferences with content that addresses the learning needs of PICU nurses, providing another avenue for continuing education. Simulation has also become an important adjunct to the training of nurses and other health care professionals. This interactive high-tech learning method is particularly appealing to the Generation-Y professionals. Another media for exchange of information is the use of Listservs for specific nursing groups or technologies. This method of networking holds great promise for those who do not have the resources to network with colleagues at a national conference.

In addition to clinical resources, socialization into practice and mentorship are important concepts now included in successful transition into nursing practice. The intent of mentoring programs is to provide socialization of the new nurse to the unit, allow for guidance in professional development, and provide support for new nurses as they transition to different phases of their practice. The mentor-mentee relationship is also important in understanding the different communication styles and values of the multigenerational workforce. The added benefit is retention when the programs work well. This is particularly important as the nursing workforce ages.

Ongoing assessment of nursing competencies is an important part of today's nursing practice. TJC requires that competency assessment be completed on the initial orientation of a new nurse and on an ongoing basis. The definition of competence has yet to be agreed upon in the literature, but generally in the clinical environment involves evaluation of skills, knowledge, and judgment as it relates to patient care and safety. Evaluation of these competencies should include not only skills required by regulatory agencies but also clinical activities that are either high risk low volume or new to clinical staff. A variety of methods have been used for validation, including skills fairs, simulation, in-services, and oral or poster presentations. An additional method of competency evaluation is certification. The AACN Certification Corporation developed a critical care certification examination Certified Critical Care Nurse (CCRN) in 1975; however, the content was most applicable to those practicing in adult critical care. The need for a pediatrics-specific examination was identified and the AACN Certification Corporation began a role delineation study in 1989 to establish the unique nature of pediatric critical care.[30,51] The pediatric CCRN examination was first held in 1992. At present, there are 2794 pediatric CCRNs nationwide (K. Harvey, personal communication, November 23, 2010).[52] In addition, there are several resources available for nurses who are preparing for the examination, including review courses, CD-ROMs, and study guides, including the AACN *Core Curriculum for Pediatric Critical Care Nursing*.[52]

The synergy model is one method used to describe nurse-patient interactions. It is the current framework for the CCRN examination. Synergy describes nursing practice based on needs and characteristics of the patient.[53] The concept is that when nursing competencies and patient characteristics are matched, synergy occurs and optimal outcomes are achieved. Patients are described based on (1) their stability, complexity, predictability, resiliency, vulnerability, and ability to participate in decision making and care and (2) resource availability. Patients in pediatric critical care units may be at the extreme ends of many of these characteristics. Nursing competencies include clinical judgment, advocacy/moral agency, caring practice, facilitator of learning, collaboration, response to diversity, systems thinking, and clinical inquiry. All these competencies play an important role in relation to patient care needs and optimal patient outcomes.

Yet another change in nursing over the last several decades is that of advanced practice roles in the PICU. Traditionally, the only advanced practice role in critical care nursing was that of the clinical nurse specialist (CNS). This master's prepared nurse was a clinical expert with expanded knowledge of nursing education, systems theory, and nursing research/quality. The role, although extremely important, was the victim of downsizing in the early 1990s, but has made a comeback as the importance of the CNS role is validated yet again. Over the last 10 years, the role of the pediatric nurse practitioner (PNP) has emerged in the PICU. The increasing number of patients seeking critical care services in combination with decreases in resident work hours has led to this rapid role emergence.[54] PNPs now provide safe, high-quality, collaborative care in many PICUs, in both private and academic care settings. In 2005, the Pediatric Nursing Certification Board validated the practice of these professionals with the institution of the Acute Care Pediatric Nurse Practitioner certification examination.[55] The role of the PNP in critical care continues to evolve as patients, technology, and the health care environment change.

THE FUTURE

In 2010, the US Congress passed and the president signed into law comprehensive health care legislation that represents the broadest changes to the health care system since the creation of the Medicare and Medicaid programs in 1965.[56] It has become increasingly more evident that by 2014, the year that the Affordable Care Act (ACA) takes effect, the health care system, although in grave danger, has the opportunity to transform its broken system to a system that could provide seamless, affordable, quality care that is accessible to all, patient and family centered, and evidence based, leading to improved health outcomes. It is not only the spiraling increase in costs or the overreliance on technology that is weighing most heavily on the US health care system but also the sheer volume of patients to be served in the very near future, approximately 32 million newly insured patients will flood the US health care system.[57]

Nurses currently comprise the largest sector of health care providers, with more than 3 million currently registered in the US, working in the frontlines of patient care; nurses are closest to the issues and thus play a vital role in helping realize the objectives set forth by the ACA. However, several barriers prevent nurses from being able to respond effectively to a rapidly changing health care environment and an evolving health care system. These obstacles must be overcome to ensure that nurses are politically poised and positioned to lead change and advance health. To address future issues, the IOM and the Robert Wood Johnson Foundation assembled an expert panel in 2008 to discuss the role of nurses in transforming the current health care system. Their prepublication report, "The Future of Nursing: Leading Change, Advancing Health," relies heavily on the evidence amassed over the last 50 years in clinical trials of the efficacy of nursing care.[57] As a result of this epic work, the committee developed 4 key messages:

1. Nurses must practice to the full extent of their education and training.
2. Nurses must achieve higher levels of education and training through an improved education system that promotes seamless academic progression.
3. Nurses must be full partners, with physicians and other health care professionals, in redesigning health care in the US.

4. Effective workforce planning and policy making require better data collection and information infrastructure.[57]

In 2001, the IOM's landmark testimony, *Crossing the Quality Chasm: a New Healthcare System for the 21st Century*, reported that health care has safety and quality problems because it relies on outmoded systems of work.[58] Today and into the future, this health care system translates into the virtual or remote ICU as a redesigned model of care using state-of-the-art technology to leverage the expertise and knowledge of intensivists and critical care nurses.[59] This model of care supports the expert bedside team in improving patient outcomes over multiple critical care units and large geographic areas. With widespread reports that intensivist-led teams and adequate nurse staffing ratios result in better patient outcomes, and with the recognition that there is a growing shortage of both, the virtual ICU model is gaining popularity as a more viable option. A virtual care delivery system presents endless possibilities for the future PICU. The future ICU care providers will take on more responsibilities as managers of care.[60] And, much like the past PICU teams and most highly developed ICU teams today, the critical care team of the future will be multidisciplinary and will function as a highly integrated team, following protocols.

It is necessary for PICU nurses to keep pace with the latest in clinical technology and develop skills to manage the plethora of new treatment methods. As patient care and family issues become increasingly more complex, so will the role of the PICU nurse.[21] Information and technology are growing at warp speed.[23] The PICU environment is being reshaped by technologies, new business models, and human needs. New PICU models will emerge haphazardly by default or coherently by design. Aspects of some sound new models are already evident in health care systems today. The future is already here.

No one group or person has the answer to the successful navigation of the future of critical care medicine and nursing. However, it is certain that there are basically 3 forces that have the potential to create a demand for ICU services in the face of a decreasing ability to meet this demand.[61] First, the aging US population. This force affects the PICU in 2 ways: an aging workforce of providers and nurses and the possibility of shifting resources from the young to the old. Second, the gap between what is possible and what is appropriate in care. Medically advanced treatments and technologies can lead to more unrealistic expectations for the families of patients in PICUs. Third, the shortages in critical care personnel are expected to get worse. Once again, critical care nurses stepped up and a partnership between the AACN, the American College of Chest Physicians, the American Thoracic Society, and the SCCM was formed to investigate the future of critical care, focusing on these challenges. This group summarized their work in a consensus document titled *Framing Options for Critical Care in the United States* (FOCCUS).[61] Their recommendations included regionalizing resources, standardizing care using practice guidelines, encouraging specialization, and restructuring the work environment. The future does not just happen. Every PICU nurse must accept responsibility for the current state, acknowledge the vision of future, and take action to place that vision into PICU nursing's future.[62]

SUMMARY

Pediatric critical care has faced many overwhelming challenges in the past that most certainly will continue in the future. In the early days of the specialty, visionary and forceful leaders dared each other to create new ways to provide care to critically ill infants and children. Nurses and physicians taught each other how to care for the smallest and most vulnerable patients in the hospital. PICUs were created from regular patient rooms and supply rooms. There is an inescapable and inevitable tension between the human factors and the PICU work environment.[4] We need to remember that although we are in the midst of tremendous shifts in health care economics and delivery, we face no greater challenges than our predecessors.[63] History helps to predict a better future. As PICU nurses continue to refine our roles, we must never lose sight of the essence of our purpose—to care for the most–at-risk children with pride and passion. Today is the time for us to rethink the way we are currently providing care in the PICU and bring that same sense of boldness from our PICU pioneers to the challenges faced in the contemporary units of today.

In 1997, the wise words of our colleagues Drs Daniel L. Levin and Frances C. Morriss (legends in the Dallas PICU world) in the preface of their book are hauntingly true today. "In the current health care climate the dynamics of hospital care may change so dramatically in the foreseeable future that children's hospitals will become centers for treatment of children either as outpatients or as intensive care patients. If this occurs, the next edition may well be entitled *Pediatric Critical Care Medicine: A Textbook of In-Patient Medicine*. Whatever the title, it will include much new information if we are permitted and encouraged by society to continue to study in the laboratory and in the hospital and to use the knowledge gained to develop even better diagnostic, monitoring, and therapeutic skills. If we are given this charge, we must also devote at least as much time and energy to understanding when to apply these skills as to how to apply them."[64] The past continues to shape the present and will most certainly be the catalyst for the future of PICU nursing.

REFERENCES

1. Pate MF. Powered by insight: pediatric intensive care nursing. AACN Adv Crit Care 2007;18(1):15–8.
2. Hardin SR, Kaplow R. Synergy for clinical excellence: the AACN synergy model for patient care. Boston: Jones & Bartlett Publishers; 2005.
3. Bratt MM, Broome M, Kelber S, et al. Influence of stress and nursing leadership on job satisfaction of pediatric intensive care unit nurses. Am J Crit Care 2000; 9(5):307–17.
4. Foglia DC, Grassley JS, Zeigler VL. Factors which influence pediatric intensive care unit nurses to leave their jobs. Crit Care Nurs Q 2010;33(4):302–16.
5. Vestal KW, Richardson K. The nature of pediatric critical care nursing: perspectives of patient, family, and staff. Nurs Clin North Am 1981;16(4):605–10.
6. Berg J. Human touch: in the complex ICU environment, critical care nurses excel at connecting with patients. 2004. Available at: http://www.nurseweek.com/ednote/04/080204_judeeberg_print.html. Accessed September 10, 2010.
7. Curley MA. The essence of pediatric critical care nursing. In: Curley MAQ, Molony-Harmon PA, editors. Critical nursing of infants and children. 2nd edition. Philadelphia: WB Saunders; 2001. p. 3–16.
8. Society of Critical Care Medicine. About SCCM: history of critical care. Available at: http://www.sccm.org/AboutSCCM/History_of_Critical_Care/Pages/default.aspx. Accessed September 10, 2010.
9. Fairman J, Kagan S. Creating critical care: the case of the hospital of Pennsylvania, 1950–1965. ANS Adv Nurs Sci 1999;22(1):63–77.
10. Zalumas J. Caring in crisis: an oral history of critical care nursing. Philadelphia: University of Pennsylvania Press; 1995.

11. Jolley J. Now and then: Florence Nightingale and children's nursing. Paedriatric Nurs 2007;19(8):12.
12. Connolly C. Growth and development of a specialty: the professionalization of child health care. Pediatr Nurs 2005;31(3):211–3, 215.
13. Fairman J, Lynaugh JE. Critical care nursing: a history. Philadelphia: University of Pennsylvania Press; 1998.
14. National Association of Children's Hospitals and Related Institutions. History of children's hospitals. Available at: http://www.childrenshospitals.net/AM/Template. cfm?Section=t&CONTENTID=12693&TEMPLATE=/CM/ContentDisplay.cfm. Accessed November 6, 2010.
15. Children's Medical Center. Available at: http://www.childrens.com/AboutUs/. Accessed November 14, 2010.
16. Epstein D, Brill JE. A history of pediatric critical care medicine. Pediatr Res 2005; 58(5):987–96.
17. Downes JJ. The historical evolution, current status, and prospective development of pediatric critical care. Crit Care Clin 1992;8:1–22.
18. American Association of Critical-Care Nurses. History of AACN. Available at: http://www.aacn.org/wd/pressroom/content/historyofaacn.pcms?menu=aboutus. Accessed September 10, 2010.
19. American Association of Critical-Care Nurses. Organizational structure. Available at: http://www.aacn.org/wd/pressroom/content/organizationalstructure.pcms?menu= aboutus. Accessed September 10, 2010.
20. Robnett MK. Critical care nursing: workforce issues and potential solutions. Crit Care Med 2006;34(3):S25–31.
21. American Association of Critical-Care Nurses. About critical care nursing. Available at: http://www.aacn.org/wd/pressroom/content/aboutcriticalcarenursing.pcms? pid=1&&menu=aboutus. Accessed September 10, 2010.
22. Levin DL. The physical setting: conceptual considerations. In: Levin DL, Morriss FC, editors. Essentials of pediatric intensive care. 2nd edition. New York: Churchill Livingston Inc; 1997. p. 1105–11.
23. Institute of Medicine. A summary of the October 2009 forum on the future of nursing: acute care. Washington, DC: The National Academies Press; 2010.
24. Hendrich A, Chow B, Skierczynski A, et al. A 36-hospital time and motion study: how do medical-surgical nurses spend their time? The Permanente Journal 2008;12(3):37–46.
25. Sensmeier J. Alliance for nursing informatics statement to the Robert Wood Johnson Foundation initiative on the future of nursing: acute care, focusing on the area of technology, October 19, 2009. Comput Inform Nurs 2010;28:63–7.
26. Tregunno D, Jeffs L, McGillis L, et al. On the ball: leadership for patient safety and learning in critical care. J Nurs Adm 2009;39(7/8):334–9.
27. Maxfield D, Grenny J, McMillan R, et al. Silence kills: the seven crucial conversations in healthcare. VitalSmarts, LC; 2005.
28. The Joint Commission. Behaviors that undermine a culture of safety. Sentinel event alert. 2008. Available at: http://www.jointcommission.org/SentinelEvents/ SentinelEventAlert/sea_40.htm?print=yes. Accessed November 15, 2010.
29. Bylone M. Healthy work environments: whose job is it anyway? AACN Adv Crit Care 2009;20(4):325–7.
30. Paterson T. Generational consideration in providing critical care education. Crit Care Nurs Q 2010;33(1):67–74.
31. AACN standards for establishing and sustaining healthy work environments: a journey to excellence. Aliso Viejo (CA): American Association of Critical-Care Nurses; 2005.

32. Fritz W. The three C's: environments where nurses thrive. Dallas (TX): Children's Medical Center; 2006.

33. Verheugt CL, Uiterwall CS, Grobbee DE, et al. Long term prognosis of congenital heart defects: a systematic review. Int J Cardiol 2008;131:25–32.

34. Feudtner C, Villareale NL, Morray B, et al. Technology-dependency among patients discharged from a children's hospital: a retrospective cohort study. BMC Pediatrics 2005;5(8). Available at: http://www.biomedcentral.com/content/pdf/1471-2431-5-8.pdf. Accessed November 24, 2010.

35. American Academy of Pediatrics. Committee on hospital care. Family-centered care and the pediatrician's role. Pediatrics 2003;112(3):691–7.

36. American College of Critical Care Medicine Task Force. Clinical practice guidelines for support of the family in patient-centered intensive care unit. Crit Care Med 2007;35(2):605–22.

37. American Association of Critical-Care Nurses. Practice alert: family presence during resuscitation and invasive procedures. Available at: http://www.aacn.org/wd/practice/content/practicealerts.pcms?menu=practice. Accessed November 20, 2010.

38. Emergency Nurses Association. Emergency nursing resource: family presence during invasive procedures and resuscitation in the emergency department. 2009. Available at: http://www.ena.org/Research/ENR/Documents/FamilyPresence.pdf. Accessed November 20, 2010.

39. Frazier A, Warren NA. A discussion of family-centered care within the pediatric intensive care unit. Crit Care Nurs Q 2010;33(1):82–6.

40. Aronson PL, Yau J, Helfaer MA, et al. Impact of family presence during pediatric intensive care unit rounds on the family and medical team. Pediatrics 2009;124:1119–25.

41. Duran CR, Oman KS, Abel JJ, et al. Attitudes toward and beliefs about family presence: a survey of healthcare providers, patients' families, and patients. Am J Crit Care 2007;16(3):270–9.

42. Petersen MF, Cohen J, Parsons V. Family-centered care: do we practice what we preach. J Obstet Gynecol Neonatal Nurs 2004;33(4):421–7.

43. Harbaugh BL, Tomlinson PS, Kirschbaum M. Parent's perceptions of nurses' caregiving behaviors in the pediatric intensive care unit. Issues Compr Pediatr Nurs 2004;27:163–78.

44. Jay SS, Youngblut JM. Parent stress associated with pediatric critical care nursing: linking research and practice. AACN Clin Issues 1991;2(2):276–84.

45. U.S. Department of Health & Human Services. The registered nurse population: findings from the 2008 national sample survey of registered nurses. Available at: http://bhpr.hrsa.gov/healthworkforce/rnsurvey/2008/. Accessed November 22, 2010.

46. Auerbach DI, Buerhaus PI, Staiger DO. Better late than never: workforce supply implications of later entry into nursing. Health Aff 2007;26:178–85.

47. Apostolidis BM, Polifroni EC. Nurse work satisfaction and generational differences. JONA 2006;26(11):306–9.

48. Keepnews DM, Brewer CS, Kovner CT, et al. Generational differences among newly licensed registered nurses. Nurs Outlook 2010;58:155–63.

49. Wilson B, Squires M, Widger K, et al. Job satisfaction among a multigenerational nursing workforce. J Nurs Manag 2008;16:716–23.

50. Lynch ME. Update from the 15th annual conference: pediatric nursing: history and possibilities. J Pediatr Nurs 2005;20(4):305–7.

51. American Association of Critical Care Nurses. Available at: http://www.aacn.org/wd/certifications/content/aboutus.pcms?menu=certification. Accessed November 22, 2010.

52. American Association of Critical-Care Nurses. Core curriculum for pediatric critical care nursing. 2nd edition. St Louis (MO): Saunders; 2006.
53. Curley MA. Patient-nurse synergy: optimizing patients' outcomes. Am J Crit Care 1998;7:64–72.
54. Molitor-Kirsch S, Thompson L, Milonovich L. The changing face of pediatric critical care medicine: nurse practitioners in the pediatric intensive care unit. AACN Clin Issues 2005;16(2):172–7.
55. Kline AM, Reider M, Rodriquez K, et al. Acute care pediatric nurse practitioners: providing quality care for acute and critically ill children. J Pediatr Health Care 2007;21(4):268–71.
56. Institute of Medicine. The future of nursing: leading change, advancing health. Prepublication copy. Washington, DC: The National Academies Press; 2010.
57. Chen PW. Nurses' role in the future of health care. The New York Times 2010. Available at: http://www.nytimes.com/2010/11/18/health/views/18chen.html?_r= 3&ref=health. Accessed November 21, 2010.
58. Institute of Medicine. Crossing the quality chasm: a new health system for the 21st century. Washington, DC: National Academy Press; 2001.
59. Myers MA, Reed KD. The virtual ICU (vICU): a new dimension for critical care nursing practice. Crit Care Nurs Clin North Am 2008;20:435–9.
60. Jerrard J. The future of critical care. The hospitalist. 2005. Available at: http://www.the-hospitalist.org/details/article/255801/The_Future_of_Critical_Care.html. Accessed November 15, 2010.
61. Dracup K, Bryan-Brown CW. Navigating the future of critical care. Am J Crit Care 2004;13:187–8.
62. Kennerly SM. Imperatives for the future of critical care nursing. Focus Crit Care 1990;17(2):123–7.
63. Connolly C. Question: why history? The U.S. in 1904: a look back. Pediatr Nurs 2005;31(2):151–2.
64. Levin DL, Morriss FC. Preface. In: Levin DL, Morriss FC, editors. Essentials of pediatric intensive care. 2nd edition. New York: Churchill Livingston Inc; 1997.

Acute Cardiac Arrhythmias Following Surgery for Congenital Heart Disease: Mechanisms, Diagnostic Tools, and Management

Linda Payne, RN, BSN[a], Vicki L. Zeigler, PhD, RN[b],*,
Paul C. Gillette, MD[c]

KEYWORDS

- Arrhythmia • Congenital heart disease • Temporary pacing
- Cardioversion • Defibrillation

Causes, contributing factors, and management of acute postoperative arrhythmias in adults are well documented. Arrhythmias are a significant cause of mortality and morbidity in adults undergoing cardiac surgery for repair of congenital heart disease (CHD)[1]; however, few data specifically address pediatric arrhythmias in the early postoperative period.[2] Potential causes of postoperative arrhythmias in children include suture placement near areas of cardiac conduction, myocardial inflammation from sutures, myocardial incisions, and an acute increase in cardiac volume and pressure.[3]

Previous studies report the incidence of cardiac arrhythmias in children during the early cardiac postoperative period as between 15% and 48%.[3–6] The risk of arrhythmia occurrence increases with younger age, longer cardiopulmonary bypass (CPB) time, increased aortic cross clamp time, and circulatory arrest or deep hypothermia.[4,5] Other predisposing factors may include cardiac muscle dysfunction, hemodynamic impairment, and electrolyte imbalances as well as pain, fever, and

The authors have nothing to disclose.
[a] Cardiac Intensive Care Unit, St Louis Children's Hospital, 1995 Graystone Dr, St Louis, MO, USA
[b] College of Nursing, Texas Woman's University, PO Box 425498, Denton, TX 76204, USA
[c] Subspeciality Services, Denton, Cook Children's Healthcare System, 209 North Bonnie Brae, Medical Building 3, Suite 100, Denton, TX 76201, USA
* Corresponding author. Cardiovascular ICU, St Louis Children's Hospital, 1995 Graystone Drive, St Charles, LA 63303.
E-mail address: vzeigler@twu.edu

Crit Care Nurs Clin N Am 23 (2011) 255–272
doi:10.1016/j.ccell.2011.04.001
0899-5885/11/$ – see front matter © 2011 Published by Elsevier Inc.

ccnursing.theclinics.com

anxiety.[7–13] Because a detailed summary of cardiac arrhythmias that can occur after surgery for CHD is beyond the scope of this article, this discussion focuses on the management of those cardiac arrhythmias most commonly seen in the immediate postoperative period. They include ventricular tachycardia (VT), ventricular fibrillation (VF), atrial flutter (AF), junctional ectopic tachycardia (JET), bradycardia, and atrioventricular block (AVB). The mechanisms of cardiac arrhythmias are reviewed followed by a brief overview of the predominant acute arrhythmias, tools used for the diagnostic evaluation of these arrhythmias, management strategies, and, finally, nursing considerations.

MECHANISMS OF CARDIAC ARRHYTHMIAS

In the immediate postoperative period, acute arrhythmia management can be challenging. To optimize patient outcomes, it is beneficial to identify the mechanism and severity of the arrhythmia with respect to overall hemodynamics and to intervene with a brisk treatment plan. The goal of these interventions is to re-establish a normal cardiac rhythm as rapidly as possible in order to avoid unwanted sequelae. Because the mechanism of the arrhythmia can be pivotal in determining the best intervention, a brief overview of those mechanisms is provided in this article, including abnormal automaticity, reentry, and triggered automaticity.

Abnormal Automaticity

Normally, automaticity occurs in specialized cardiac electrical cells of the conduction system or the atrial muscle. The components of the conduction system are the sinoatrial node (SAN), the atrioventricular node (AVN), the bundle of His, the left and right bundle branches, and the Purkinje system.[14] During normal sinus rhythm, the propagation of each electrical impulse terminates after the atria and ventricles have been activated. The SAN, which possesses these specialized cells of automaticity, must spontaneously generate a new impulse for the cycle of excitation and propagation to begin again. Once activated (depolarization), cardiac tissue cannot be reactivated until it has nearly reached its resting state (repolarization). During the time between depolarization and repolarization, the tissue is described as refractory. Refractory is the time in which the cardiac tissue cannot respond to external stimuli and depolarize.

Cardiac automaticity is defined as spontaneous impulse initiation, the excitation of which is propagated from cell to cell resulting in depolarization across the myocardium.[15] Automaticity is an inherent property of the SAN. Abnormal automaticity occurs when cardiac tissue becomes irritated and overtakes the normal rates of the SAN. In tissue that does not have intrinsic automaticity, abnormally rapid rates may occur. These rhythms are modulated by the autonomic nervous system and demonstrate hallmark characteristics, such as a variation of rate manifested as a gradual onset and gradual termination of the tachycardia. The increased sympathetic tone associated with recovery from surgery, inotropic support, and/or fever often accentuates this type of arrhythmia.

Automatic tachycardias are known to originate from atrial muscle, the area of the bundle of His or bundle branches, and ventricular muscle.[16] The most common automatic arrhythmias that occur in the immediate postoperative period (discussed later) are JET and VT. Atrial fibrillation is much less common than other arrhythmias in the pediatric population but may be due to abnormal automaticity,[17] but because of its rarity in children, it is not discussed in this article. Automatic rhythms demonstrate a higher incidence of diminished responsiveness to medication and neither overdrive pacing nor direct current shock is effective in terminating the arrhythmia.

Reentry

In some circumstances, abnormal conduction is propagated around a boundary. The boundary can be anatomic, such as a scar, nodal tissue, and/or a band of tissue connecting the atria to the ventricle, or the boundary can be functional, such as diseased or injured tissue. In order for reentry to occur, 3 coexisting factors must be present. There must be 2 distinct but adjacent pathways. The pathways must have a difference in conduction rates, and there must be unidirectional block in one of the pathways.[16] Of the 2 pathways, there is a fast pathway and a slow pathway. The fast pathway has a shorter conduction time and a longer refractory time, whereas the slow pathway has a longer conduction time and a shorter refractory period. Typically, electricity travels down the slow pathway whereas the fast pathway is refractory. The completion of the cycle down one pathway and up the other pathway initiates reentrant tachycardia.

Reentrant tachycardia can occur in the atrium, in the AVN, through a band of tissue connecting the atrium and the ventricle at either the tricuspid valve or mitral valve (atrioventricular), or in the ventricles. Reentry may be exhibited in single beats or sustained runs of tachycardia. The hallmark characteristics of reentrant tachycardia are that (1) the rapid rate does not vary, (2) the episodes occur paroxysmally (or intermittently), and (3) the onset and termination of the tachycardia is abrupt. Reentrant rhythms commonly seen in the immediate period after surgery for CHD that are discussed include AF and VT. Overdrive pacing and/or direct current cardioversion are effective in terminating reentrant arrhythmias and medication management is more likely to be efficacious.

Triggered Automaticity

Triggered automaticity is a conceptual idea. In vitro studies have demonstrated that triggers are comprised of oscillations in the cell membrane. These oscillations increase the cellular voltage, which exceeds the membrane threshold potential and causes a premature beat. The premature beat creates more oscillations causing more beats and eventually causing a triggered rhythm, which is manifested in a polymorphic tachycardia.[18] This concept is strongly associated with torsades de pointes and linked to long QT syndrome. It is more difficult to identify triggered automatic rhythms because the hallmark signs mimic both abnormal automaticity and reentry. These rhythms mimic automaticity in that there may be a varying rate with gradual onset and termination. Medication management is less effective for triggered as it is in automatic rhythms. Triggered automaticity imitates reentry in that it is more amenable to overdrive pacing or cardioversion.[16]

ARRHYTHMIA OVERVIEW

Supraventricular tachycardia (SVT) is a broad category of arrhythmias that includes atrial tachycardia, AF, and JET. Owing to the fact that these arrhythmias can originate anywhere above the bifurcation of the bundle of His, they generally exhibit the same QRS complex on the surface ECG as that of sinus rhythm. The P waves are often not visible or are hard to discern due to the rapid ventricular rate. Additional testing may be required to differentiate the type of SVT. The most common form of SVT in the acute postoperative period is JET, which originates in the AV junction area, in particular the bundle of His. In a study of 28 of 189 pediatric patients who had undergone surgery for CHD, more than half of them exhibited JET.[4] The ECG on patients with JET demonstrates narrow, rapid QRS complexes without visualization of P waves or difficult to identify P waves (**Fig. 1**).

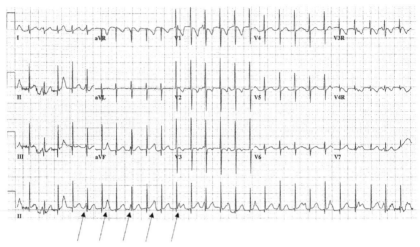

Fig. 1. JET. 15-Lead ECG from a 13-month-old with junctional ectopic tachycardia. Note the presence of a narrow QRS tachycardia with AV dissociation (dashed arrows depicting P waves in one segment of the ECG), where the ventricular rate is faster than the atrial rate.

AF is also a reentrant circuit within the atrial muscle. AF is less common in the immediate postoperative period but is common as a chronic arrhythmia in children and adults with CHD.[19] With AF, the ECG demonstrates sawtooth pattern morphology with respect to the P waves, also known as flutter waves, with QRS complexes that may or may not be regular (**Fig. 2**). The flutter waves conduct to the ventricle in a variable manner (see **Fig. 2**). With atrial fibrillation, the ECG demonstrates intermittent QRS complexes and a fine chaotic atrial rhythm between the QRS complexes (**Fig. 3**).

VT is defined as a rapid ventricular rhythm most likely initiated by a reentrant circuit within the ventricles.[20] It can be diagnosed on the ECG by the presence of a wide complex tachycardia that is different from that of sinus rhythm and that has dissociation between the ventricles and atria (**Fig. 4**). In the postoperative setting, it can be responsible for tachycardia-induced cardiomyopathy, significant hemodynamic impairment, and sudden death.[16] VF is a rapid quivering of the ventricular muscle, which does not produce any cardiac output. It is fatal without immediate intervention.[20] The ECG reveals no formed P waves or QRS complexes and rapid undulating waveforms may be present (**Fig. 5**).

Sinus bradycardia is a slowing of the sinus node to below normal rates. The ECG demonstrates a normal complex QRS that is preceded by a P wave; however, the rate is below what is considered normal based on age-related and situation-related criteria. Various degrees of AVB can be seen in children in the immediate postoperative period. The AV node may be sluggish or incapable of conduction from the atria to the ventricles. Consequently, there may be prolonged AV conduction (first-degree AVB), intermittent AV conduction (second-degree AVB), or a complete block in conduction (third-degree AVB) (**Fig. 6**).[20]

TOOLS FOR DIAGNOSTIC EVALUATION

Although it is not always possible to differentiate arrhythmias based on their mechanisms, it is helpful to distinguish arrhythmias based on common characteristics and behaviors.[20] In critical situations, a clinician must be able to discern the type of

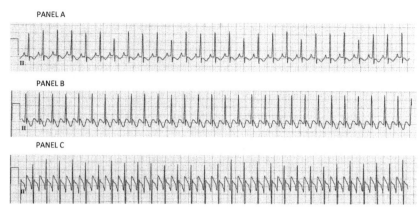

Fig. 2. AF. Rhythm strip tracings in lead II from an 11-month-old girl with complex CHD and postoperative AF. (*A*) Baseline tracing demonstrating a narrow QRS rhythm at 163 bpm. P waves appear to precede each QRS and that T waves are inverted. (*B*) 4 Hours later after an increase in heart rate to 176 bpm, T waves continue to be inverted but P waves are lost. The baseline is now reminiscent of a sawtooth pattern. (*C*) An atrial electrogram using a temporary atrial pacing lead. The diagnosis of AF with a 2:1 ventricular response is now confirmed.

arrhythmia quickly and intervene in order to prevent further deterioration of the rhythm and preserve hemodynamic stability of the patient. There are several tools available to assist in the diagnosis of early postoperative arrhythmias.

Telemetric Monitoring

Telemetry is a useful tool used to continuously observe rhythms.[21] Although a rhythm strip is not used to diagnose hypertrophy or ischemia, advanced telemetry systems

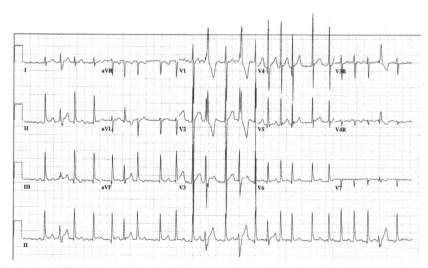

Fig. 3. Atrial fibrillation. 15-Lead ECG from a 12-year-old male with palpitations demonstrating atrial fibrillation with a variable ventricular response. Irregular baseline highlights the lack of coordinated atrial activity. The occasional wide QRS beats with a right bundle branch block morphology. These likely represent aberrant conduction due to right bundle refractoriness.

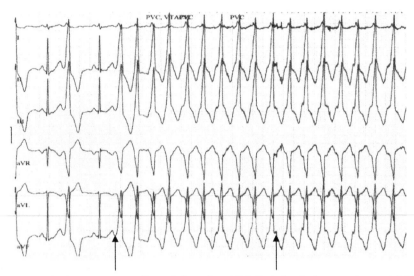

Fig. 4. VT. Rhythm strip recording of 6 surface ECG limb leads in a patient exhibiting bigeminal PVCs during normal sinus rhythm followed by the onset of monomorphic VT. In leads III and aVF, dissociated P waves can be seen preceding or just after the widened QRS complex (*arrows*).

can provide helpful information in the form of graphic data regarding average heart rates, associated oxygen saturation levels, and blood pressure trends as well as hemodynamic markers, such as central venous pressures. Lead II is the most common lead used in rhythm strips because the P wave and QRS complexes are clearly detectable the majority of the time. The use of telemetric monitoring is standard while patients are in an ICU and is largely used on cardiac units during postoperative recovery. If a rhythm strip seems to have changed either in timing cycles or in waveform, an ECG strip should be recorded for clinician evaluation.

ECG

The ECG enables a rhythm to be assessed in multiple leads rather than in a single lead.[21] The ECG assists in visualizing a clear P wave and a QRS complex, which

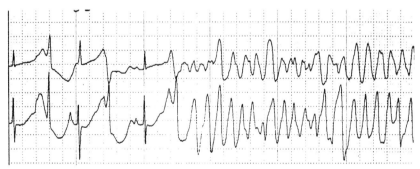

Fig. 5. VF. Rhythm strip recording of 2 surface ECG leads demonstrating a markedly prolonged QT interval with T wave alternans that degenerates into a form of VF known as torsades de pointes.

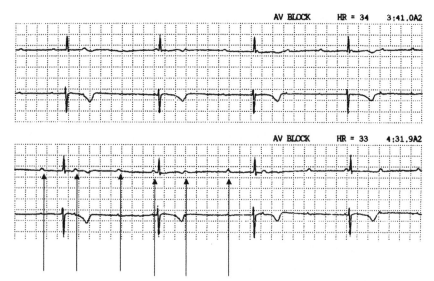

Fig. 6. Complete AVB. Rhythm strip recording of 2 surface ECG leads in a patient with complete (third-degree) AVB with a narrow QRS complex. The P waves (*arrows*) have no relationship to the QRS complexes indicating the complete absence of AV conduction.

can be measured. It also provides additional information regarding the axis of the P wave and the QRS complex. Diagnoses of hypertrophy, ischemia, and abnormal activation patterns can be made from an ECG. The heart rate can be interpreted as fast or slow and the rhythm as regular or irregular. The QRS is wide or narrow based on patient age. If the rhythm is wide and rapid, VT should be presumed until proven otherwise.[16] An ECG should of the presenting rhythm should be obtained unless the patient is too hemodynamically unstable or clearly are in VF. In that situation, the ECG should be deferred. After each intervention for the arrhythmia, a rhythm strip recording is sufficient. When the rhythm is restored to sinus, a final ECG should be performed.

Temporary Epicardial Pacing Wires

Temporary epicardial pacing wires are commonly placed in the operating room after congenital heart repair.[22] Although the wires are not used regularly, they can be used as an expedient method for cardiac pacing. The complexity of the pacing wires varies. A bipolar configuration is by far the preferred polarity; however, their placement should be conducted in a manner in which they are easy to remove. Because bradycardia and its variants are unpredictable in the postoperative setting, at least 2 atrial and 2 ventricular wires should be placed at the time of surgery. If the bradycardia is of sinus or junctional origin, atrial pacing alone should restore an adequate rate and improve hemodymanics. In the case of second-degree or third-degree AVB, atrioventricular (or dual chamber) pacing likely provides the best rate support and hemodynamic benefit. If complete AVB (CAVB) is a likely result of the repair in certain complex congenital heart lesions, consideration should be given to placing both right and left ventricular pacing wires, lending to the use of biventricular pacing.

Epicardial wires can be used as a diagnostic aide or as treatment modality or both for various arrhythmias.[23] The wires are used to (1) provide rate support for bradyarrhythmias, such as sinus and junctional bradycardia; (2) enhance atrioventricular synchrony during various degrees of AVB; (3) overdrive reentrant tachyarrhythmias, such as SVT or AF; and (4) aide in the differential diagnosis of arrhythmias. To overdrive pace an atrial, junctional, or ventricular reentrant tachycardia, a cycle length (in milliseconds) versus a rate (in beats per minute [bpm]) that is 70% of the tachycardia cycle length is an initial starting point for overdrive pacing. Burst pacing of 8 to 32 beats can be used; however, the faster the pacing rate that is used, the more likelihood there is of inducing an arrhythmia that results in increased hemodynamic compromise.

The origin of a narrow complex tachycardia may be difficult to determine. Connecting atrial and ventricular wires to a recording system enables identification of the chamber initiating the rhythm. Additionally, with the occurrence of JET, epicardial atrial wires can be used by pacing incrementally faster than the junctional rate, providing atrioventricular synchrony.[22] Use of epicardial wires for pacing is not a singular therapy but should occur simultaneously with pharmacologic interventions in an effort to restore patients to normal sinus rhythm.

Esophageal Electrograms

When atrial activity cannot be clearly identified on a surface ECG, an esophageal catheter may be used.[24] A depth chart based on patient height is used to determine the length of the catheter that must be inserted into the esophagus through the mouth or nares to achieve a prominent atrial electrogram. The tip of the catheter has sensing and pacing electrodes and is inserted via the esophagus and positioned behind the atrium. This improves detection of atrial activation and promotes atrial pacing and capture. This use of this tool requires a pacing cart with cardiac electrogram recording capabilities. The purpose of esophageal pacing is similar to that of temporary epicardial pacing with the exception of ventricular pacing. The esophageal catheter can be used for arrhythmia differentiation as well as overdrive pacing of reentrant tachycardias, such as SVT or AF. If the catheter is used to pace, it is recommended that patients receive analgesia because pacing in the esophagus can cause severe discomfort.

Permanent Pacemaker/Defibrillator Interrogation

In the event that patients with a permanent cardiac pacemaker or implantable cardioverter defibrillator have undergone repair for CHD and are experiencing arrhythmias, the device may be interrogated and used to differentiate rhythms as well as to overdrive pace and eradicate the arrhythmia.[25,26] Diagnostic data stored within the device and recordings of intracardiac electrograms can assist clinicians in making diagnostic or management decisions by virtue of interrogating the device. The implantable cardioverter defibrillator in particular can be programmed for overdrive pacing for termination of stable VT and low-dose cardioversion for hemodynamically stable AF, atrial fibrillation, and/or VT.

MANAGEMENT OF POSTOPERATIVE ARRHYTHMIAS

The urgency in the management of arrhythmias in the postoperative period is based on a patient's hemodynamic status and, in part, by the mechanism of the arrhythmia. If the mechanism of the arrhythmia is unclear, a clinician may use the diagnostic tools (discussed previously) to identify the rhythm abnormality. Multiple modalities may be used in the treatment of these arrhythmias. The hemodynamic status of patients largely determines in what order these modalities are implemented. The treatment modalities include (1) pharmacologic therapy and/or (2) electrical therapy.

Pharmacologic

Pharmacologic therapy is used for the treatment of both bradyarrythmias and tachyarrhythmias (**Table 1**). During the immediate postoperative period, these drugs are administered intravenously (IV). The most common medications used in the immediate postoperative period discussed in this article include adenosine, amiodarone, atropine, digoxin, esmolol, isoproterenol, lidocaine, and procainamide. There is a cadre of antiarrhythmic agents used in children with cardiac arrhythmias that are not discussed; the ones discussed are those that are commonly used in acute instances of arrhythmia occurrence.

Adenosine

Adenosine is a class IV antiarrhythmic agent.[27] It is used to terminate a variety of reentrant arrhythmias and to assist in the differential diagnosis of various substrates of SVT, such as atrioventricular nodal reentry tachycardia (AVNRT) versus SVTs with concealed bypass tracts versus AF.[28] It is also effective in terminating substrates of SVT, such as concealed bypass tracts and AVNRT.[28] Adenosine is rapidly metabolized[16] and consequently has an extremely short half-life (ie, <10 seconds).[29] Therefore, to increase efficacy, administration should occur in a central vessel/line if possible or in a large peripheral vein immediately followed with a bolus of saline.

Adenosine acts by reducing impulse formation of the sinus and AVN and by slowing conduction through the AVN. This disrupts the reentrant circuit and terminates SVTs, which rely on the AVN for continuation of the arrhythmia. Therefore, when adenosine is given during narrow complex tachyarrhythmias, those tachycardias that do not rely on the AVN are not terminated. For example, in children with AF, the administration of adenosine reveals AF waves as it blocks conduction in the AVN. As a reentrant atrial muscle tachycardia, AF does not rely on the AVN for perpetuation; therefore, it is not terminated with adenosine. Potential adverse effects of adenosine include exacerbation of asthma, chest pressure, facial flushing, headache, lightheadedness, nausea, transient complete heart block, and/or diaphoresis.[27] If patients are aware of their surroundings, they should be made aware of the potential adverse effects and assured that they are transient. Adenosine is not a long-term treatment modality. If adenosine is effective in terminating the SVT, another medication should be loaded and given to maintain normal sinus rhythm. Additionally, when adenosine is used, a form of ventricular pacing should be readily available at the bedside in the event that the bradycardia or ventricular asystole that commonly occurs with its administration is not transient. Arrhythmias that are not amenable to adenosine include atrial tachycardias that are due to an automatic focus, AF, atrial fibrillation, JET, and VT.

Amiodarone

Amiodarone is a class III antiarrhythmic agent. Its primary functions are to prolong cardiac tissue refractoriness and suppress automaticity. Amiodarone depresses automaticity in the SA and AV nodes and slows conduction diffusely throughout the heart.[30] It is predominantly used to treat atrial and ventricular arrhythmias that have not responded to other medications. Postoperative arrhythmias that are particularly amenable to amiodarone are AETs, JET, and VT.[31,32] Recently, the American Heart Association (AHA) pediatric advanced life support (PALS) guidelines recommended amiodarone administration as the preferred treatment for pulseless VT and VF.[33]

Nurses caring for patients receiving IV amiodarone must be knowledgeable regarding potential adverse effects and drug interactions. Acutely, IV amiodarone can cause hypotension. The optimal form of measuring blood pressure while amiodarone is loaded is via arterial catheter placement. Because cardiac tissue refractory

Table 1
Common pharmacologic agents used for acute postoperative arrhythmias

Agent	Dosage	Cardiovascular Contraindications	Other Pertinent Information
Adenosine	Bolus: 100–150 µg/kg given rapid IV push followed quickly with saline flush; double dose sequentially to maximum of 300 µg or the adult dose of 6–12 mg	• Prolonged QT interval • Second- or third-degree AVB, except in presence of temporary/permanent pacing • Sick sinus syndrome	• Have defibrillator available when administering, in event of ventricular rate acceleration, torsades de pointes, or VF • Caffeine makes adenosine less effective • Avoid use in patients with asthma due to bronchoconstriction effects • Use with caution in patients receiving digoxin • Incompatible with any drug in solution or syringe.
Amiodarone	Bolus: 5 mg/kg (1 mg/kg over 5 minutes) OR 2.5 mg/kg given twice Infusion: 10–15 mg/kg/d	• Sick sinus syndrome except in presence of temporary/permanent pacing • AVB, except in presence of temporary/permanent pacing • Cardiogenic shock	• Monitor blood pressure, heart rate, and rhythm continuously • Transient hypotension can be treated with volume or calcium chloride infusion • Due to vasodilatory effects, may potentiate effects of certain antihypertensives
Atropine	IV/IO: 0.02 mg/kg ET: 0.04–0.06 mg/kg Repeat once as needed Minimum dose: 0.1 mg Maximum single dose: 05 mg[33]	• Tachyarrhythmias • Asthma • Myocardial ischemia • Acute hemorrhage	• May be given endotracheally and intraosseously • May cause paradoxic bradycardia in infants, especially with slow IV administration • Not stable in alkaline solutions • Helpful in patients with vagally mediated bradycardia • Helpful for bradycardia/AVB in patients with neurologic injuries • Monitor ECG for heart rate and rhythm continuously

Drug	Dosing	Comments
Digoxin	Total digitalizing dose: Premie infant: 20 µg/kg Full-term newborn: 30 µg/kg Infants <2 years: 40–50 µg/kg Children >2 years: 30–40 µg/kg Maintenance dose: 25% of total digitalizing dose every 12 hours	• Hypertrophic obstructive cardiomyopathy (may worsen outflow obstruction) • WPW (may enhance accessory pathway conduction; in presence of AF with rapid conduction, may result in VF) • AVB except with pacemaker • Unrepaired tetralogy of Fallot • Renal dysfunction can prolong digoxin half-life for as long as 1 week • Digoxin toxicity more likely if hypokalemic or hypercalcemic • Monitor heart rate, rhythm, and PR interval constantly • Monitor serum potassium, magnesium, and calcium in select patients
Esmolol	Loading: 500 µg/kg over 1–2 minutes Maintenance: 50–200 µg/kg/min	• Sinus bradycardia, second- or third-degree AVB except with temporary or permanent pacing • Cardiogenic shock • Heart failure • Use with caution in patients with ↓renal function, diabetes, or bronchospasm • Effects subside within 2–3 minutes, complete reversal in 30 minutes • Solution is incompatible with diazepam, furosemide, sodium bicarbonate, and thiopental sodium • Recommended for short term use only (<48 hours) • Avoid extravasation (very acidic solutions can lead to skin necrosis)
Isoproterenol	Initial dosing: 0.05–1.0 µg/kg/min (increase infusion rate every 5 minutes until desired effect seen) Continuous Infusion: 20–50 µg/kg/min	• Presence of myocardial ischemia • Arrhythmias secondary to digoxin toxicity • Causes ↑in pulse pressure characterized by ↓in diastolic and ↑in systolic pressure • Continuous ECG monitoring • Increases myocardial oxygen consumption • Drug decomposes rapidly in alkaline solutions

(continued on next page)

Table 1
(continued)

Agent	Dosage	Cardiovascular Contraindications	Other Pertinent Information
Lidocaine	Loading dose: 1 mg/kg every 5 minutes × 3 doses Continuous infusion: 20–50 µg/kg/min	• Severe sinus and AVN dysfunction without pacemaker	• Can be administered ET and IO • Continous ECG monitoring • Use decreased dose in patients with congestive heart failure or liver failure • Serum concentrations range from 2–5 µg/mL • Monitor potassium levels—more effective with higher potassium levels • Reduce dose when using with halothane
Procainamide	Loading dose: Infants: 7–10 mg/kg over 30–45 minutes Older children: bolus of 15 mg/kg Infusion: 40–50 µg/kg/min (infants occasionally need up to 100 µg/kg to maintain therapeutic serum concentration)	• Second- or third-degree AVB without pacemaker • Torsades de pointes • Congestive heart failure • Prolonged QT interval	• Decrease dose when patient also receiving cimetidine • Continuous ECG monitoring • Monitor serum concentration of procainamide (4–8 µg/mL) and NAPA (10–30 µg/mL) • NAPA is active metabolite of procainamide • Monitor potassium levels (↓ level may lead to ↑arrhythmias)

Abbreviations: ET, endotracheally; IO, intraosseously; NAPA, *N*-acetylprocainamide; WPW, Wolff-Parkinson-White syndrome.
Adapted from Knick BJ, Saul JP. Immediate arrhythmia management. In: Zeigler VL, Gillette PC, editors. Practical management of pediatric cardiac arrhythmias. Armonk (NY): Futura Publishing Co, Inc; 2001. p. 189–95; with permission.

periods are longer and conduction is slower on amiodarone, there is a high incidence of a prolonged QT interval during loading. Various degrees of AVB also may occur. This may be particularly true in patients who have undergone congenital heart repair and have an injured conduction system. Therefore, a temporary means of ventricular pacing should be available at the bedside. Patients should be continuously monitored by ECG and receive a daily ECG with measurement of the QT and PR intervals.

Multiorgan toxicity is a known adverse effect of amiodarone; however, these affects generally occur with long-term use. The particular organs affected are the eyes, lungs, liver, and thyroid. Corneal deposits may accumulate on the eyes. The lungs may become fibrotic, the liver may demonstrate elevated enzymes leading to cirrhosis or hepatitis, and hyperthyroidism/hypothyroidism may occur.[27] Thus, for chronic amiodarone administration, baseline ophthalmic, pulmonary function, liver enzyme, and thyroid function tests must be obtained. If amiodarone becomes a long-term therapy, these tests must be done every 6 months.

Finally, clinicians should be aware that amiodarone may potentiate other drug levels to the point of toxicity. The most noted interaction is with digoxin. Studies have shown that when digoxin is given concurrently with amiodarone, there is a 25% to a 100% rise in serum digoxin concentrations.[34] Before amiodarone is initiated, the current digoxin dose should be decreased by 33% to 50% to avoid digoxin toxicity.[34] There is a significant interaction between amiodarone and warfarin (Coumadin). Prothrombin and internationalized normalized ratios should be monitored frequently when patients are receiving both of these pharmacologic agents.

Atropine

Atropine sulfate is classified as an anticholinergic agent. Its purpose in the postoperative setting is to treat symptomatic bradycardia. It increases heart rate and conduction velocity as a result of decreased vagal tone. Arrhythmias responsive to atropine are symptomatic sinus bradycardia and vagally induced bradycardia. Because atropine improves bradycardias, which originate above the ventricles, it is not effective in resolving advanced or complete AVB. Nurses caring for patients receiving atropine must be aware of the potential vagal response associated with its use, which can cause profound bradycardia if less than 0.01 mg/kg is given.[27] The AHA recommends a minimum dose of 0.1 mg/kg.[33] The potential side effects of atropine are tachycardia, dry mouth, flushed skin, dilated pupils, hypotension, and hypertension. Older children who may be awake might be able to feel the symptoms and should be forewarned of their potential occurrence.

Digoxin

Digoxin is classified as a cardiac glycoside. It enhances myocardial function and is used to suppress or terminate reentrant tachycardias by slowing conduction through the AVN. Arrhythmias that use the AVN as part of their circuits includes concealed bypass tracts and AVNRT.[30] Digoxin can also used in patients with AF and atrial fibrillation to slow AVN conduction and alleviate the possibility of 1:1 conduction of the arrhythmia; it can also be used to create AVB for the same purpose, both of which serve to slow the ventricular rate and improve hemodynamics.[30] Digoxin can be given to patients who experience JET to decrease the risk of heart failure. The potential adverse reactions associated with digoxin administration are nausea, vomiting, and drowsiness. Presence of these symptoms suggests cardiac toxicity along with conduction disturbances, such as second-degree or third-degree AVB. When this occurs, obtaining a digoxin serum concentration is recommended.

Esmolol

Esmolol hydrochloride is a class II antiarrhythmic. It is a β-blocker also known to have a short half-life. Additionally, esmolol increases systemic vascular resistance and decreases cardiac contractility. The β-blocker effects occur primarily in the atrial muscle and the SA and AV nodes. The sinus rate slows, the recovery period prolongs, and the conduction through the AVN slows. The effect is a decreased heart rate as well as diminished cardiac contractility. Esmolol is often used to treat tachyarrhythmias after surgical repair of congenital heart disease.[35,36] Arrhythmias that particularly respond to esmolol are reentrant SVTs, AVNRT, JET, AF, and VT. Because esmolol can decrease myocardial function, it should be avoided in patients with heart failure, and precaution should be taken in giving it to patients with decreased ventricular function. The risk for acute hypotension in young children is significant and in those with single ventricle physiology.[34] For that reason, patients receiving esmolol should have continuous cardiac and blood pressure monitoring, preferably with an arterial line rather than an external blood pressure measurement. Slower administration of the dose is recommended if patients exhibit bradycardia and/or hypotension.

Isoproterenol

Isoproterenol is a pure β-adrenergic agonist. In the postoperative setting, it is used primarily to treat hemodynamically compromising bradycardia caused by sinus node dysfunction or AVB.[33] It is also used as a ventricular rate support for patients who have acquired advanced or complete heart block and are waiting for permanent pacemaker implantation.[27] There is an increase in conduction velocity, heart rate, myocardial contractility, and vasodilation.[30] Common adverse affects include palpitations, chest pain, headache, nausea, and vomiting.

Lidocaine

Lidocaine is classified as a 1B antiarrhythmic agent (sodium channel blocker). It is used primarily as a local anesthetic. Postoperatively, however, its principal use is for management of ventricular arrhythmias. Its action is directed toward the ventricles and it has little effect on the sinus or AV node. Lidocaine reduces spontaneous ventricular ectopy by interrupting the reentrant circuit around scarred or diseased tissue. The use of lidocaine may indirectly lower defibrillation thresholds, which, in turn, may make it easier to terminate VF.[30] Arrhythmias that are amenable to lidocaine are premature ventricular contractions (PVCs) and VT. Nurses caring for patients receiving lidocaine should be aware that it can be proarrhythmic (arrhythmia inducing). It can also exacerbate certain forms of SVT. As the drug is being administered, continuous ECG rhythm monitoring should be available. Clinicians should observe for decreased ventricular ectopy. Adverse reactions include soreness at the site of IV insertion and alterations in mental status or level of consciousness. Somnolence and confusion may be indicative of toxicity and if not recognized quickly may lead to seizures.[27]

Procainamide

Procainamide is classified as a 1a agent. It works by slowing generalized conduction in the atrium, His bundle, and ventricle. It directly slows AVN conduction, which is more pronounced as the heart rate increases.[30] Abnormal rhythms, which respond well to procainamide, are SVTs with the substrate of concealed bypass tracts, AVNRT, AF, atrial fibrillation, PVCs, and VT. Patients should be continuously monitored for new-onset arrhythmias or for blood pressure, especially hypotension. If new arrhythmias or exacerbation of the offending arrhythmia occurs, a physician should be contacted and the medication discontinued. The chief adverse effect is hypotension. Arterial blood pressure should be monitored closely. Because AVN conduction is slowed, some form of temporary pacing should be available in the event that advanced heart block occurs.

Electrical

Electrical interventions used in the management of postoperative arrhythmias include synchronized cardioversion, external defibrillation, intracardiac electrophysiology studies and ablations, and pacemaker and defibrillator implantation. These treatment modalities are specialized and designed to terminate tachyarrhythmias or to prevent bradyarrhythmias.

Direct current cardioversion

The purpose of synchronized direct current cardioversion is to convert unstable SVT or VT to sinus rhythm. Synchronized cardioversion delivers an electrical shock via transthoracic pads or paddles, which depolarize enough of the myocardium so that the remainder of cardiac tissue is unable to sustain the arrhythmia. The shock is synchronized to the ventricular intrinsic activity. When the defibrillator is set to synchronized mode, the machine detects each QRS wave and delivers an electrical shock during ventricular depolarization. If the machine is not in sync mode and the shock is delivered during ventricular repolarization, VF may occur.

Arrhythmias that are receptive to direct current cardioversion are AF, atrial fibrillation, reentrant SVTs, and reentrant VT. Automatic rhythms, such as atrial ectopic tachycardias and JET, are not amenable to cardioversion. Synchronized cardioversion can be used in two separate circumstances. It can be used electively to stop AF or atrial fibrillation or it can be used more emergently to terminate unstable SVT or VT. In preparation for synchronized cardioversions of either type, an IV must be in place for the purpose of delivering resuscitation drugs. Cardioversion is a painful experience if patients are awake. Therefore, if patients are not too unstable, time should be taken to administer sedation. There should be continuous ECG monitoring along with continual oxygen saturation measurements. Blood pressure should be monitored throughout the procedure. Patients who have undergone surgical repair for CHD may have an increased risk of significant bradycardia following cardioversion.[30] A means of external pacing should be available. External defibrillators are capable of using the stimulation pads to pace.

The AHA PALS guidelines recommend the appropriate paddle/pad size based on age and body weight[33] (ie, adult-sized [8–10 cm] for children >10 kg and infant-sized for infants <10 kg). There are 2 options for pad placement. The first is to place the paddle/pad anterior/posterior. The front pad should be placed directly over the heart and the back pad is placed over the right posterior hemithorax. The second option is the anterior pad placed in the upper right chest below the clavicle and the other pad placed at the apex.[33] If patients have a pacemaker or defibrillator, the pads/paddles should be placed as far away as possible from the device. The stimulation pads are self-adhesive and contain conductive gel. When paddles are used, conductive gel should be applied. Gels used for echocardiograms are not acceptable because they conduct electricity poorly.[30] The pads/paddles must be intact to avoid arcing of electricity and chest burns.

The AHA guidelines recently updated the recommendation on the dosage for cardioversions to 1 J/kg to 2 J/kg of body weight[33] and low-dose energy via shocks that use biphasic waveforms have been successful in terminating atrial arrhythmias in children and adults with and without CHD.[37] Rhythms that are less organized require more energy for conversion.[33] It is optimal for patients to be placed on nothing by mouth for at least 4 hours before the procedure. If patients are unstable, the cardioversion should be done regardless of patient nutritional status.

External defibrillation

External defibrillation is similar to synchronized cardioversion; however, the shock is not synchronized to the QRS complex. Defibrillation is an untimed depolarization of energy, which stuns the myocardium and allows time for the initiation of an organized beat, optimally originating from the sinus node.[30] The arrhythmias responsive to defibrillation are pulseless VT, VF, or torsades de pointes. These rhythms do not have an organized QRS complex and, therefore, cannot be synchronized. The PALS guidelines also updated the defibrillation dosage to 2 J/kg to 4 J/kg of body weight.[33] Peak doses of amiodarone increase defibrillation thresholds.[30] If patients are on amiodarone, successful defibrillation may require a higher starting dose. After defibrillation, the areas covered by the stimulation pads or paddles should be examined for burns or abrasions.

NURSING CONSIDERATIONS

Nursing care of pediatric postoperative surgical patients can be challenging. Nurses must be aware of physiologic processes, changing hemodynamic status, impact of medications and interventions on the arrhythmia, and the psychodynamics of patients and families. Nurses should recognize a postoperative rhythm and intervene swiftly if hemodynamic status is compromised. If feasible, patients and families should be informed about the rhythms, their impact on patients, and interventions required to terminate the arrhythmia. This should be done in an age-appropriate language to facilitate comprehension. In stressful situations, patient and family understanding may fluctuate.[30] Information should be repeated multiple times and in various ways to facilitate understanding. With the addition of medications, the nurse must perform a careful assessment before and after medication administration. Familiarity with patient status enhances recognition of a change in a patient's condition. Any change in status should be communicated to a physician. For any procedure done at the bedside, nurses should be familiar with the process and be able to recognize any adverse effects. Aside from being a care provider, a nurse is often a communication liaison. Therefore, a nurse should ensure that patient and family are well prepared for any upcoming procedures. Nurses should collaborate with the multidisciplinary team to provide appropriate teaching and education for patients and families. For any intervention that creates a lifestyle change after discharge from the hospital, patients and families should be made aware and given time to process the information. There should be transparency between patients and the medical and nursing staff in order for patients and families to develop trust in the team.

Pediatric patients exhibiting arrhythmias after repair of a congenital heart defect demands astute observation and rapid intervention. Nurses should be knowledgeable regarding the surgical repair, the mechanisms responsible for the arrhythmia, the availability of tools for diagnosis of the arrhythmia, and the types of interventions used to terminate the arrhythmia.

REFERENCES

1. Yueh-Tze L, Lee J, Wentzel G. Postoperative arrhythmia. Curr Opin Cardiol 2003; 18:73–8.

2. Kertesz NJ, Friedman RA, Fenrich AL, et al. The incidence of perioperative arrhythmias. In: Balaji S, Gillette PC, Case CL, editors. Cardiac arrhythmias after surgery for congential heart disease. New York: Arnold; 2001. p. 50–63.

3. Valsangiacomo E, Schmid ER, Schupback RW, et al. Early postoperative arrhythmias after cardiac operation in children. Ann Thorac Surg 2002;74:792–6.

4. Delaney J, Moltedo J, Dziura JD, et al. Early postoperative arrhythmias after pediatric cardiac surgery. J Thorac Cardiovasc Surg 2006;131:1296–300.

5. Rekawek J. Risk factors for cardiac arrhythmias in children with congenital heart disease after surgical intervention in the early postoperative period. J Thorac Cardiovasc Surg 2007;133:900–4.

6. Pfammatter JP, Wagner B, Berdat P, et al. Procedural factor associated with early postoperative arrhythmias after repair of congenital heart defects. J Thorac Cardiovasc Surg 2002;123:258–62.

7. Pfammatter JP, Bachmann DC, Bendicht PW, et al. Early postoperative arrhythmias after open-heart procedures in children with congenital heart disease. Pediatr Crit Care Med 2001;2:217–22.

8. Garson A Jr, Gillette PC. Junctional ectopic tachycardia in children: electrocardiography, electrophysiology and pharmacologic response. Am J Cardiol 1979;44:298–302.

9. Hoffman TM, Wernovsky G, Wieand TS, et al. The incidence of arrhythmias in a pediatric cardiac intensive care unit. Pediatr Cardiol 2002;23:598–604.

10. Hoffman TM, Bush DM, Wernovsky G, et al. Postoperative junctional ectopic tachycardia in children: incidence, risk factors, and treatment. Ann Thorac Surg 2002;74:1607–11.

11. Walsh EP, Saul JP, Sholler GF, et al. Evaluation of a staged treatment protocol for rapid automatic junctional tachycardia after operation for congenital heart disease. J Am Coll Cardiol 1997;29:1046–53.

12. Satur CMR, Stubington SR, Jennings A, et al. Magnesium flux during and after open heart operations in Children. Ann Thorac Surg 1995;59:921–7.

13. Dormann BH, Sade RM, Burnette JS, et al. Magnesium supplementation in the prevention of arrhythmias in pediatric patients undergoing surgery for congenital heart defects. Am Heart J 2000;139:522–8.

14. Moorman AF, de Jong F, Denyn MF, et al. Development of the cardiac conduction system. Circ Res 1998;82:629–44.

15. Spooner PM, Rosen MR. Foundations of cardiac arrhythmias: basic concepts and clinical approaches. New York: Marcel Dekker, Inc; 2001.

16. Walsh EP, Saul JP, Triedman JK, et al. Cardiac arrhythmias in children and young adults with congenital heart disease. Philadelphia: Lippincott Williams and Wilkins; 2001.

17. Haissaguerre M, Jais P, Shah D, et al. Spontaneous initiation of atrial fibrillation by ectopic beats originating in the pulmonary veins. N Engl J Med 1998;339:659–66.

18. Rosen M, Wit A. Triggered activity. In: Zipes D, Rowlands D, editors. Progress cardiol arrhythmias part III. Philadelphia: Lea & Febiger; 1998. p. 39–46.

19. LeRoy S, Dick M II. Supraventricular arrhythmias. In: Zeigler VL, Gillette PC, editors. Practical management of pediatric cardiac arrhythmias. Armonk (NY): Futura; 2001. p. 53–109.

20. Woods LS, Sivarajan Froelicher ES, Underhill Motzer S. Cardiac nursing. 4th edition. Philadelphia: JB Lippincott; 2000:583, 839.

21. Zeigler VL, Marlow D, Gillette PC. Mechanisms, diagnostic tools, and patient and family education. In: Zeigler VL, Gillette PC, editors. Practical management of pediatric cardiac arrhythmias. Armonk (NY): Futura; 2001. p. 1–52.

22. Ceresnak SR, Pass RH, Starc TJ, et al. Predictors for hemodynamic improvement with temporary pacing after pediatric cardiac surgery. J Thorac Cardiovasc Surg 2011;141(1):183–7.

23. Moltedo JM, Rosenthal GL, Delaney J, et al. The utility and safety of temporary pacing wires in postoperative patients with congenital heart disease. J Thorac Cardiovasc Surg 2007;134:515–6.

24. Cohen MI, Vetter VL. Postoperative atrioventricular conduction defects. In: Balaji S, Gillette PC, Case CL, editors. Cardiac arrhythmias after surgery for congenital heart disease. New York: Arnold; 2001. p. 85–118.

25. Taylor SJ, Zeigler VL, Clark JM. Permanent pacemakers. In: Zeigler VL, Gillette PC, editors. Practical management of pediatric cardiac arrhythmias. Armonk (NY): Futura; 2001. p. 305–58.

26. Zeigler VL, Corbett K, Lewis A, et al. Implantable cardioverter defibrillators. In: Zeigler VL, Gillette PC, editors. Practical management of pediatric cardiac arrhythmias. Armonk (NY): Futura; 2001. p. 359–407.

27. Turkoski BB, Lance BR, Tomsik EA, editors. Drug information handbook for advanced practice nursing. Hudson (OH): Lexi-Comp; 2009. p. 55–7.

28. Wren C. Adenosine in paediatric arrhythmias. Paediatr Perinat Drug Ther 2006; 7(3):114–7.

29. Ratnasamy C, Rossique-Gonzales M, Young ML. Pharmacological therapy in children with atrioventricular reentry: which drug? Curr Pharm Des 2008;14:753–61.

30. Knick BJ, Saul JP. Immediate arrhythmia management. In: Zeigler VL, Gillette PC, editors. Practical management of pediatric cardiac arrhythmias. Armonk (NY): Futura Publishing Co, Inc; 2001. p. 189–95.

31. Perry JC, Fenrich AL, Hulse JE, et al. Pediatric use of intravenous amiodarone: efficacy and safety in critically ill patients from a multicenter protocol. J Am Coll Cardiol 1996;27(5):1246–50.

32. Lane RD, Nguyen KT, Niemann JT, et al. Amiodarone for the emergency care of children. Pediatr Emerg Care 2010;26(5):382–9.

33. Kleinman ME, Chameides L, Schexnayder SM, et al. Part 14: pediatric advanced life support: 2010 American Heart Association Guidelines for Cardiopulmonary Resuscitation and Emergency Cardiovascular Care. Circulation 2010;122(Suppl 3): S876–908.

34. Perry JC. Medical antiarrhythmic therapy. In: Gillett PC, Garson A Jr, editors. Clinical pediatric arrhythmias. 2nd edition. Philadelphia: WB Saunders Company; 1999. p. 231–48.

35. Esmolol Research Group. Intravenous Esmolol for the treatment of supraventricular tachyarrhythmia: results of a multicenter, baseline controlled safety and efficacy study in 160 patients. Am Heart J 1986;112:498–505.

36. Trippel DL, Wiest DB, Gillette PC. Cardiovascular and antiarrhythmic effects of Esmolol in children. J Pediatr 1991;119(1):142–7.

37. Liberman L, Hordof AJ, Altmann K, et al. Low energy biphasic waveform cardioversion of atrial arrhythmias in pediatric patients and young adults. Pacing Clin Electrophysiol 2006;29:1383–6.

Use of Continuous Glucose Monitoring Systems in Children with Type 1 Diabetes

Pantea P. Minnock, RN, MSN, CRNP, CCRP*,
Carol J. Howe, RN, MSN, CNS, CDE

KEYWORDS

• Child • Type 1 diabetes • Glucose monitoring systems

Diabetes is one of the most common chronic illnesses in children and adolescents, with approximately 151,000 people younger than 20 affected.[1] Each year, more than 15,000 children, ie, 40 per day, are diagnosed with Type 1 diabetes in the United States.[2] The incidence of Type 1 diabetes is rising in children, with a change from 13.3/100,000 persons per year in 1990 to 14.6 in 2000,[3] suggesting a continual upward trend.

The Diabetes Control and Complications Trial (DCCT) was a landmark study confirming for the first time that maintaining near normal glucose levels decreased the risk of long-term complications associated with diabetes.[4] Intensive management reduced the risk of retinopathy by 76%, of microalbuminuria by 39%, and of clinical neuropathy by 60%. Because of these findings, there has been a greater emphasis on intensive diabetes treatment with the goal of maintaining increasingly tighter diabetes control and lower A1c levels as a child grows and matures.[5]

Intensive diabetes management requires that children and parents monitor blood glucose, count carbohydrates, and administer insulin via injection or pump at least 4 times a day. In addition, they must constantly consider the interplay among insulin, food, and activity to make treatment decisions that balance the goal of near-normal blood glucose levels with the risk of hypoglycemia. One consequence of tighter diabetes control is a marked increase in the frequency of hypoglycemia.[6]

Naturally, patients and parents, especially parents of younger children who may not perceive the onset of hypoglycemia, fear the risk of a severe hypoglycemic episode.

The authors have nothing to disclose.
Department of Endocrinology, Diabetes Center for Children, The Children's Hospital of Philadelphia, 34th and Civic Center Boulevard, Philadelphia, PA 19104, USA
* Corresponding author.
E-mail address: minnockp@email.chop.edu

Crit Care Nurs Clin N Am 23 (2011) 273–290
doi:10.1016/j.ccell.2011.04.004
0899-5885/11/$ – see front matter © 2011 Elsevier Inc. All rights reserved.

Studies have found that parents have great fear and anxiety for their children as they strive for near-normal blood glucose levels with this known risk for more frequent episodes of hypoglycemia.[7,8] Parental fear of hypoglycemia was associated with higher HbA1c levels and higher frequency of problematic hypoglycemic events in the past year.[9] Anxious about hypoglycemia, parents check their child's blood glucose frequently, avoid being away from their child, and feed their child at the slightest sign of low blood glucose.[8] Additionally, older children and adolescents who do much of their own self-care may also fear hypoglycemia. Adolescents who had a severe hypoglycemic episode with loss of consciousness had significantly higher A1c levels after the event.[10]

Nocturnal hypoglycemia, associated with lower baseline A1c levels, is of particular concern. Approximately one-third of parents report monitoring their child's blood glucose frequently during the night; the frequency of nighttime blood glucose monitoring was associated with increased parental anxiety and stress.[11] The Juvenile Diabetes Research Foundation Continuous Glucose Monitoring study found that hypoglycemic events occurred with the median of 7.4% of nights per subject with hypoglycemia episodes lasting 2 or more hours on 23.0% of the nights when hypoglycemia occurred.[12]

Continuous glucose monitoring systems (CGMS) offer a recent technological solution to fear of hypoglycemia. With glucose readings every 5 minutes, and the alarm capabilities to signal rapid increases or decreases in blood glucose, they afford a sense of security for both children and parents. Although children and parents must continue to be vigilant in the treatment of diabetes, CGMS may effectively allow tight diabetes control with earlier detection of hypoglycemia onset. This article provides an overview of CGMS available at the time of publication; new generations of systems have been introduced annually with improvements in sensitivity and user friendliness.

CGMS—WHAT IT IS/WHAT IS AVAILABLE

The advent of CGMS, aka glucose sensors, is revolutionary in the clinical and everyday management of children with Type 1 diabetes. Referred to as the "third era" in diabetes management,[13] these devices provide users with nearly continuous data on glucose variability. Families now have a way to track glucose levels throughout the day and night.

CGMS works by measuring glucose levels in the interstitial fluid. The CGMS is commonly placed on the upper buttocks or abdomen but can also be worn on an arm or leg. The device consists of 3 separate components. The first component of the system is a sensor-a flexible, thin, disposable catheter that is inserted subcutaneously using an inserter unit to ensure accurate depth and angle of insertion. A needle introduces the sensor underneath the skin and is retracted, leaving a thin plastic or stainless steel catheter. The tip of the catheter contains a glucose oxidative enzyme that reacts with the glucose in the interstitial fluid, generating an electric signal; the higher the signal, the higher the amount of glucose detected and vice versa (**Fig. 1**). This electrical signal is converted to a blood glucose reading through a calibration process using self blood glucose monitoring.[14] The sensor is backed with an adhesive pad that keeps it adhered to the skin. A glucose value is generated every 1 to 5 minutes depending on the specific device.

The second component of the CGMS is the transmitter, which is a compact electronic device that attaches to the top of the skin adhesive/sensor unit. The transmitter receives the electrical signal from the sensor and wirelessly communicates the information to

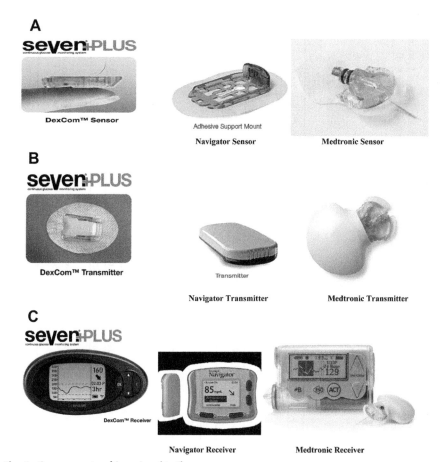

Fig. 1. Components of imaging (A–C).

a receiver, the third portion of the device system, on which the glucose data appear and are stored. The main screen of the receiver typically displays the current glucose value, a graph depicting recent trends, and predictive arrows providing information on the direction and rate of glucose change. Users are able to view up to 24 hours of information directly on the receiver with the use of trend graphs. Through the receiver, the patient calibrates the system using a standard blood glucose measurement, programs the device (eg, set alarm thresholds), and flags information related to daily activities (ie, times/amount of insulin administration, activity, food consumption).

Each CGMS has corresponding data management software to upload the data stored in the receiver for retrospective analysis of glucose patterns and trends. In the United States, there are currently 4 sensors that are commercially available for patient personal use: (1) Abbott Freestyle Navigator (Abbott Park, IL, USA), (2) Dexcom SEVEN PLUS (San Diego, CA, USA), (3) MiniMed Paradigm Revel REAL-Time, and (4) MiniMed Guardian REAL-Time (Northridge, CA, USA). Only 2 sensors, the MiniMed Paradigm and Guardian, are approved for use in the pediatric population (ie, age 7 years and older); however, off-label use is common practice. **Table 1** provides a comparison of these devices.

Table 1
Comparison of available continuous glucose monitoring systems

System	FreeStyle Navigator (Abbott)	Dexcom SEVEN PLUS (Dexcom)	REAL-Time Guardian (Medtronic MiniMed)	REAL-Time Revel System (Medtronic MiniMed)
Picture				
Approval for Use – Age	18 yrs old +	18 yrs old +	7 yrs old +	7 yrs old +
Approval for Use – Length of Wear	5 days	7 days	3 days (anecdotal report of 6+ days)	3 days (anecdotal report of 6+ days)
Glucose Data	Every 1 minute	Every 5 minutes	Every 5 minutes	Every 5 minutes
Trend Graphs	Yes – 2, 4, 6, 12, 24 hour graphs	Yes – 1, 3, 6, 12, 24 hour graphs	Yes – 3, 6, 12, 24 hour graphs	Yes – 3, 6, 12, 24 hour graphs
Rate of change information	Yes	Yes	Yes	Yes
Alarms for hyper and hypoglycemia	Yes	Yes	Yes	Yes
Calibration	Direct – receiver is also a glucometer	Manual	Manual	Modified Direct
Sensor Size & Insertion	21 Gauge 5mm length Straight (90°)insertion	26 Gauge 13mm length Angled (45°)insertion	23 Gauge 13mm length Angled (45°)insertion	23 Gauge 13mm length Angled (45°)insertion
Data Management Software	Freestyle CoPilot	Dexcom Data Manager	Carelink Personal	Carelink Personal
Cost	$1450 (device) $450 for pack of 6 $75 per sensor	$999 (device) $316 for pack of 4 sensors $79 per sensor	$1199 (device) $145 for pack of 4 sensors $36.25 per sensor	$999 (device after cost of pump) $350 for pack of 10 sensors $35 per sensor
Product Website	www.freestylenavigator.com	www.dexcom.com	www.minimed.com/products/guardian	http://www.minimed.com/products/insulinpumps

BENEFITS OF USING CGMS

CGMS provides a volume of information regarding glucose variability that has never been possible before. Users can now see the impact of multiple entities-eg, food, exercise, and stress-on glucose levels. All CGMS sensors provide a minimum of 288 glucose readings per day compared with the recommended minimal testing of 4 times a day (before meals and bedtime). With the additional data from CGMS, users can identify personal patterns and trends in hyperglycemia and hypoglycemia that are often missed with routine blood glucose checks.

CGMS use has been shown to positively affect patient outcomes by increasing the amount of time spent in euglycemia.[15–20] CGM simultaneously improves control, as measured by lower hemoglobin A1C levels, and decreases episodes of hypoglycemia, which typically rise with tightened control.[21]

CGMS use in children has been shown to significantly reduce glycemic variability, controlling extreme rises or falls in blood glucose.[17] Garg and colleagues[16] demonstrated that patients using CGMS spent 21% less time hypoglycemic, 23% less time hyperglycemic, and 26% more time in their target range compared with control subjects who used traditional blood glucose monitoring.

Features of the CGM device, such as trend graphs, alarms/alerts, and predictive arrows/alerts, are able to warn users of impending hyperglycemia and hypoglycemia, providing an opportunity for timely action and lifestyle modification to reduce occurrence. This information can be seen in real time and can also be reviewed retrospectively, allowing for multiple points of data analysis. Analysis of the data can help users (and caregivers of the users) to modify insulin regimens, activity, and diet (such as carbohydrate amount and type) to improve glycemic control.

A key benefit of sensor use is the ability to identify and prevent hypoglycemia.[22] These devices have been used to study the prevalence of hypoglycemia with results indicating that (1) hypoglycemia is common in children with diabetes, (2) children are often asymptomatic during hypoglycemic excursions, and (3) blood glucose checks at bedtime are poor predictors of hypoglycemia during the night.[23–25] Rates of hypoglycemia, especially nocturnal hypoglycemia, are better identified and duration is reduced with CGM in comparison with standard blood glucose testing.[25,26] Fear of hypoglycemia is a major factor preventing good diabetes control and can be alleviated with use of glucose sensors. Case Study 1 (Appendix 1) illustrates a child with missed overnight hypoglycemia.

Another benefit of CGM is the ability to evaluate glucose rise after meals.[19] Significant postprandial hyperglycemia excursions, especially after the breakfast meal, have been identified in children with diabetes contributing to elevated hemoglobin A1C levels.[24] CGMS captures the rate and duration of blood glucose increase after eating. Alarms can be set to signal hyperglycemia. Patients can modify their diets and the timing/amount of insulin administered to improve postprandial blood glucose. Case Study 2 illustrates a child with postprandial hyperglycemia.

CGM is a valuable tool for evaluating the impact of exercise on glycemic control.[27] Because most children are typically very active, parents worry about how glucose levels are affected by physical activity. The risk for nocturnal hypoglycemia is greater after a day of heavy exercise or activity.[28] CGM results can be used in real time to manage acute episodes of hypoglycemia and hyperglycemia during exercise, as well as to detect a decreasing blood glucose trend. Retrospective review from the device software can be used to determine the effect of different activities on glucose levels.

Several clinical trials have identified frequency of use as a key component in achieving the benefits of CGM.[29–31] In the largest trial to date on the use of CGMS in adults and children, the Juvenile Diabetes Research Foundation (JDRF) found that subjects who used the system more than 5 days a week achieved a better hemoglobin A1C level and increased time in euglycemia than those who wore it less consistently.[31] These results were found during the 6-month original trial, and were confirmed in the 6-month extension arm of the trial.[32] Although only 20% of the pediatric subjects, ages 8 to 17 years, were able to sustain high-frequency use at the end of 12 months, this group experienced the greatest improvement from baseline A1C levels.[33]

BARRIERS PREVENTING USE OF CGMS

In our diabetes center, we have seen that motivation and interest in CGM use is initially very high but decreases over time. This reduction in use has been identified in several studies, including the JDRF Continuous Glucose Monitoring Trial[33] and the DirectNet Study Group.[17] Considering that the frequency of use is directly correlated with the degree of benefit that the device users experience, it is critical to identify barriers to use.

One of the main problems if CGMS use is inconsistent accuracy and reliability of the device. Families get frustrated that blood glucose can sometimes vary by more than 50 points from a sensor reading. To understand this phenomenon, it is essential to keep in mind that glucose in the interstitial fluids (ISF) is not the same as blood/plasma glucose.[34] Glucose in the ISF is a fraction of that found in the blood. Furthermore, diffusion and equilibration between the two (from ISF to blood and vice versa) takes time. This concept of physiologic lag time results in a mismatch between the blood glucose and the sensor glucose readings. The difference can be 10% to 20% at any given time and is more pronounced during rapid rises or falls in blood glucose. Unfortunately, accuracy and reliability is most problematic during times of hypoglycemia.[14] Because of these reasons, clinicians must educate patients that it is not advisable to make management decisions based solely on the CGMS readings. A standard blood glucose measurement, via fingerstick, is necessary before giving insulin, or treating hyperglycemia or hypoglycemia.

Frequent false alarms are another barrier to consistent CGM use. Users become dissuaded from using the device when alarms (both high and low) are interfering with daily activities.[27] For children, alarms can be a source of embarrassment when triggered in public areas, such as school or sporting events. To increase accuracy and to reduce the frequency of false alarms, users are taught to calibrate at times when blood glucose is stable to improve the correlation between CGM and blood glucose measurements. However, calibrating CGM and blood glucose readings during periods of minimal glucose variation can be a challenging task in children because of their varied and inconsistent eating and activity patterns.[35]

Educators from the DirectNet Navigator Pilot study identified insertion and skin problems as the most unanticipated difficulty with sensor use. The problems users experienced were (1) sensor not inserting properly, (2) too much bleeding during insertion, (3) accidental dislodging of sensor, (4) sensor not sticking well to skin, and (5) development of skin rash/irritation from the sensor adhesive.[36] Issues with tape and adhesives are particularly troublesome for children who typically have less body surface and subcutaneous tissue than their adult counterparts.[37]

Unrealistic expectations of both children and their parents can lead to disappointment and discontinuation of CGM. Patients and families naively believe that this technology will reduce the amount of work involved in their diabetes management.[38] Many are hopeful that CGM is a magic replacement for time-consuming and often uncomfortable standard blood glucose monitoring. Instead, families learn that CGM requires intensive management.

The emotional response to one's "naked" diabetes, because all glucose variability is identified and recorded, can be complex and overwhelming, resulting in users opposing device use.[39] The constant feedback on glucose levels can be a source of stress for both parents and children. Adolescents are particularly sensitive to this, as CGM use has the potential to violate their privacy by serving as the "glucose tattle," magnifying dietary/lifestyle indiscretions and poor management choices.[27,35]

A major challenge in CGM use is high cost and poor insurance coverage.[38] Although improvement in coverage has occurred over the past few years, many are still unable to meet the financial responsibilities associated with frequent sensor use.[40]

PATIENT EDUCATION

A well-developed educational program is essential for promoting the successful use of CGM. The first step in the education process is identifying candidates who are likely to use the system, therefore benefiting from all that the device offers. The JDRF trial found that age (>25 years old), frequency of blood glucose monitoring before study enrollment, and amount of CGM use in the first month of initiation were predictive of long-term use.[41]

The American Association of Clinical Endocrinologists (AACE) has recently released a consensus panel on continuous glucose monitoring.[40] They recommend real time/personal CGM for patients who experience frequent hypoglycemia, hypoglycemia unawareness, an above-target A1C level, and excessive glycemic variability. Additionally, for CGM use in children and adolescents, the AACE recommends choosing candidates who are likely to use the device. Successful candidates are those who frequently monitor blood glucose, have an A1C of less than 7%, and are highly motivated. Those whose A1C is greater than 7% can also be successful candidates if they agree to use the device almost daily.

Additional factors to consider in choosing candidates include physical stature (does the user have enough subcutaneous fat to accommodate sensor use), stable diabetes regimen (so that stress is reduced), strong diabetes support system (to share the responsibility of device use), individual motivation (child interest in addition to parental interest), and ability to afford the technology.[27,33,35]

The core of the educational program should be directed toward helping families choose the device that best meets their needs and subsequently preparing them for the reality of CGM use. It is important to present both the benefits and limitations of this technology to set realistic expectations.[27,35,38,39,42,43] Education should emphasize that CGM does not replace regular blood glucose testing and should not be used as the only means of alerting patients to low or high glucose values. Additionally, sensor values should never be used to make clinical decisions on the amount of insulin administration and when to treat hypoglycemia or hyperglycemia.

The clinician and the child/family should discuss the common barriers to CGM use and strategies to reduce potential discouragement. Because accuracy and reliability are greatly increased with optimal calibration, the clinician can review a child's typical day to help families choose appropriate calibration times. Problems with false alarms can be minimized by teaching users to appropriately set alarms and the methods to maximize responses when they are triggered. By setting more liberal alarms initially to improve tolerability, the clinician can work with the child and parent to raise the threshold to a higher level once glucose variability has improved. Skin problems should be managed aggressively with early identification and treatment with different tapes and skin barriers to reduce discomfort.

Attention to the developmental and psychosocial needs of children is important. Toddlers/preschoolers will be less involved in the decision-making process but older children, and especially adolescents, should be in agreement with their parents regarding initiation and use of the device. Families should be encouraged to take a nonjudgmental approach to the data and view glucose excursions as information to make treatment decisions. Although clinicians, patients, and parents can become mired in the glucose data, it must be remembered that the goal is to balance quality of life with improvements in glycemic control.

After CGM initiation, providers should periodically review the benefits/barriers of device use with their patients to proactively determine what may be limiting use and to work with families to minimize problems. Those who have Internet access will benefit from the resources available; the user manual for each device is publically accessible, as are demonstration videos of setting up the system, insertion/removal of sensors, calibration, and troubleshooting of alarms. Please see **Table 2** for online resources related to CGM.

Continuing education after CGM initiation should focus on empowering families to manage and respond to the volume of information generated in both real-time and retrospective reviews of data. A thorough review on the basics of diabetes management with an emphasis on insulin function and mechanism of action is necessary to prevent problems, such as insulin stacking and overtreatment of lows.[35,40] The DirectNet Applied Treatment Algorithm (DATA) has been developed as a guideline to help users make management decisions using glucose values and has been shown to be both feasible and user friendly.[44] Educating families about the use of this algorithm can help increase confidence and independence in making insulin adjustments.

FUTURE OF CGM

The ultimate goal of technology in diabetes management is a closed loop system (artificial pancreas) where euglycemia can be achieved through a multihormonal pump system integrated with a glucose monitoring system. The advent of CGMS has served to make this goal more achievable than ever before. Roadmaps to achieve this goal are recommended by field experts such as Dr Aaron Kowalski.[45]

At present, the CGM system is only an adjunct to traditional blood glucose monitoring. The technology of these devices is still in its infancy and numerous limitations prohibit full integration in standard diabetes management. Brauker[46] identified 5 goals for device development that are necessary to widen adoption of CGM in the broader population: (1) improved reliability, (2) ease of use, (3) comfort, (4) integration with other products, and (5) affordability. The immediate future of device development should focus on improving device safety and efficacy so that CGM data can be used as the primary source of information for decision making.[46]

The American Association of Clinical Endocrinologists[40] recommends the following aims for future CGM product development: (1) improved blood glucose–reading

Table 2
Web sites with information regarding continuous glucose monitoring systems

Name	Web Address	Content
Children with Diabetes	www.childrenwithdiabetes.com/continuous.htm www.childrenwithdiabetes.com/cgm.htm	• CGMS Comparison Chart • Link to scientific research studies on CGM • Blogs with information from families using CGM • Article for families about what CGM is and expectations of use
Diabetes Health	www.diabeteshealth.com/browse/products/cgms/	• CGMS Reference Guide • Articles related to CGM use—listed in chronologic order with latest info appearing at top of page
Jaeb Center for Health Research (JCHR)—Continuous Glucose Monitoring School	https://studies.jaeb.org/ndocs/extapps/CGMTeaching/Public	• Online CGM School – tutorial on use and function of CGMS. Includes device-specific case studies & modules
American Association of Clinical Endocrinologists	http://alt.aace.com/pub/pdf/ContinuousGlucoseMonitoring.pdf	• AACE consensus statement on continuous glucose monitoring (Released September 2010)
Diabetes Mall	www.diabetesnet.com/diabetes_technology/continuous_monitoring.php	• Comparison chart on current CGMS • Information on future devices under development
Tu Diabetes	www.tudiabetes.org/group/cgmusers www.tudiabetes.org/forum/categories/continuous-glucose-monitoring/listForCategory	• Discussion forum & support groups for users of CGMS

accuracy; (2) development of a single-platform intuitive software that combines information from CGM devices, meters, and pumps, (3) integration of personal CGM device/meters, pumps; (4) integration and connectivity of CGM with insulin pumps and pens; and (5) CGM algorithms that are proactively responsive to the rate of glucose change. Future research recommendations include focusing on long-term studies to assess efficacy and durability, cost-effectiveness, best candidates for CGM, and continued product development to refine the accuracy and comfort of the devices.

Research targeted at CGM use in children has been limited to date, but designing and conducting such trials to assess CGM efficacy is a priority.[43] Only 2 of the 4 available devices in the United States are indicated for use in the pediatric population. Clinical trials assessing short-term and long-term efficacy in the pediatric population are necessary. More information is needed on how these devices work in children and how the unique needs of this population can be met with CGM use.

SUMMARY

In summary, CGMS have the ability to revolutionize the management of Type 1 diabetes. The potential for benefit is vast and includes the ability to improve glycemic control by preventing and reducing periods of hypoglycemia and hyperglycemia. A key benefit for children is the ability to identify glucose excursions during sleep, after eating, and with exercise. The advantages of CGM are directly correlated with the frequency of device use. Barriers to use include problems with accuracy and reliability, false alarms, comfort/skin problems, unrealistic user expectations, psychosocial impact, and cost. Successful use of CGM can be promoted by identifying ideal candidates and implementing a comprehensive educational program that sets realistic expectations and addresses the unique needs of children. The future of CGM research and product development should be directed toward improving the system to make the ultimate goal of diabetes technology—a closed loop system—achievable.

APPENDIX 1

Case Study 1: Nocturnal Hypoglycemia

A 4-year-old child on multiple daily injection regimen of NPH and Humalog insulin. First morning blood glucoses are typically in range or elevated. Sensor results reveal that child experiences prolonged hypoglycemia (<40 mg/dL) on several nights that are not detected as blood glucose rises in the early morning hours. Timing and dose of NPH insulin was changed after this sensor trial to minimize overnight hypoglycemia. Parents were educated on checking overnight blood glucose periodically, especially on high-activity days.

Case Study 2: Postprandial Hyperglycemia

A 7-year-old child with positive pancreatic antibodies and glucose intolerance had previously been able to maintain normal glycemic control without insulin therapy. Sensor results reveal adequate fasting glucose and postprandial hyperglycemia. Hyperglycemia is most pronounced after the breakfast meal. Insulin therapy was started after sensor trial.

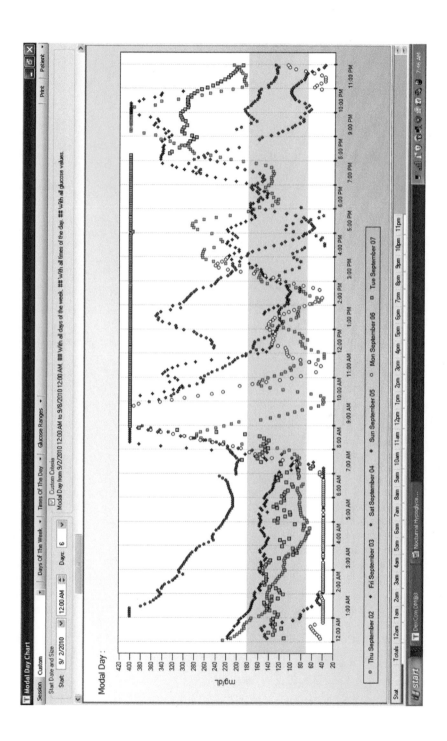

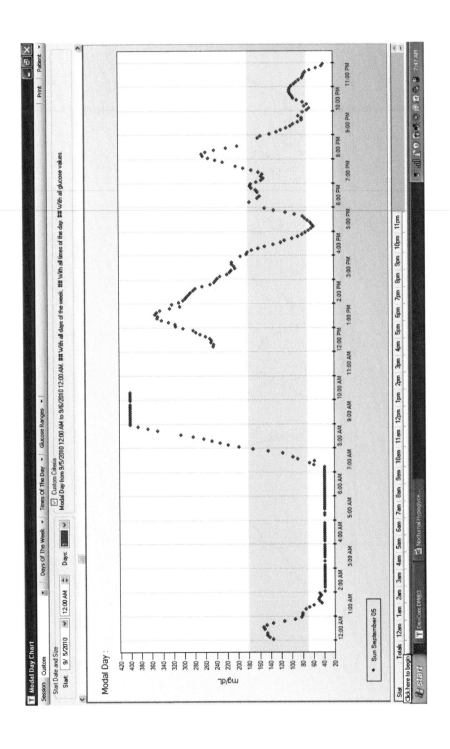

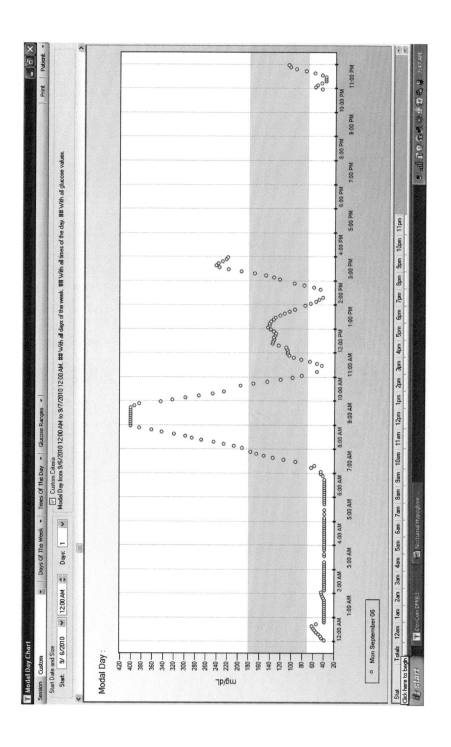

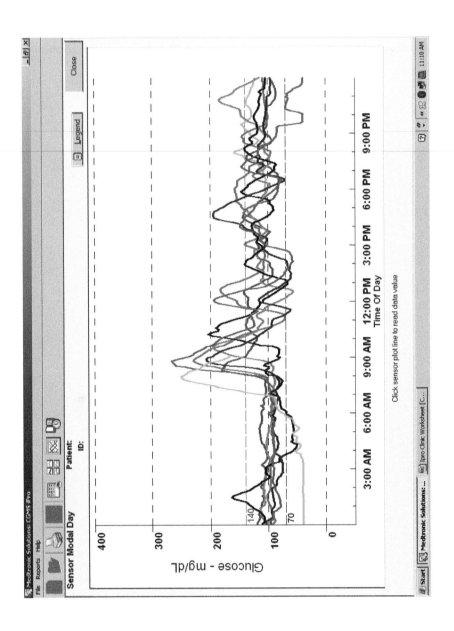

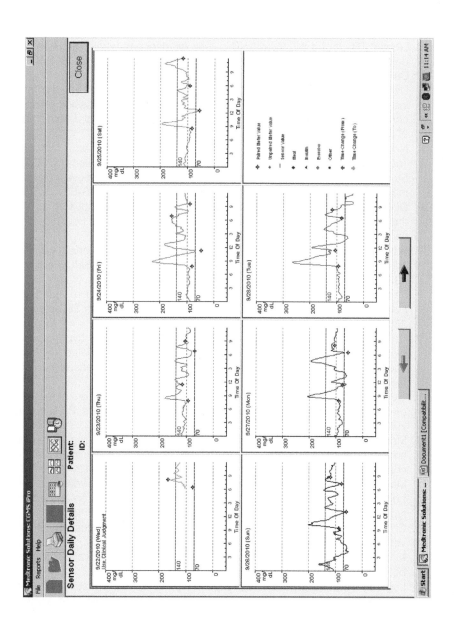

REFERENCES

1. Centers for Disease Control and Prevention (CDC). Children and diabetes—more information. 2010. Available at: http://www.cdc.gov/diabetes/projects. Accessed November 13, 2010.
2. Juvenile Diabetes Research Foundation. Type 1 Diabetes (Juvenile Diabetes) Facts. 2010. Available at: http://www.jdrf.org. Accessed November 13, 2010.
3. Lipman TH, Jawad AF, Murphy KM, et al. Incidence of type 1 diabetes in Philadelphia is higher in black than white children from 1995 to 1999. Diabetes Care 1999;29(11):2391–5.
4. Diabetes Control and Complications Trial Research Group. The effect of intensive insulin treatment of diabetes on the development and progression of long-term complications on insulin-dependent diabetes mellitus. N Engl J Med 1993;329: 977–85.
5. Nathan DM, Cleary PA, Backlund JY, et al. Diabetes Control and Complications Trial/Epidemiology of Diabetes Interventions and Complications (DCCT/EDIC) Study Research Group. Intensive diabetes treatment and cardiovascular disease in patients with type 1 diabetes. N Engl J Med 2005;353:2643–53.
6. Diabetes Control and Complications Trial Research Group. Adverse events and their association with treatment regimens in the diabetes control and complications trial. Diabetes Care 1995;18:1415–27.
7. Barnard K, Thomas S, Royle P, et al. Fear of hypoglycaemia in parents of young children with type 1 diabetes: a systematic review. BMC Pediatr 2010; 10:50–8.
8. Patton SR, Dolan LM, Powers HR. Parental fear of hypoglycemia: young children treated with continuous subcutaneous insulin infusion. Pediatr Diabetes 2007;8: 362–8.
9. Haugstved A, Wentzel-Larsen T, Graue M, et al. Fear of hypoglycaemia in mothers and fathers of children with type 1 diabetes is associated with poor glycaemic control and parental emotional distress: a population-based study. Diabet Med 2010;27:72–8.
10. Gonder-Frederick LA, Fisher CD, Ritterband LM, et al. Predictors of fear of hypoglycemia in adolescents with type 1 diabetes and their parents. Pediatr Diabetes 2006;7:215–22.
11. Monaghan MC, Hillard ME, Cogen FR, et al. Nighttime caregiving behaviors among parents of young children with type 1 diabetes: associations with illness characteristics and parent functioning. Fam Syst Health 2009;27(1):28–38.
12. Mauras N, Xing D, Beck RW, et al. Prolonged nocturnal hypoglycemia is common during 12 months of continuous glucose monitoring in children and adults with type 1 diabetes. Diabetes Care 2010;33(5):1004–15.
13. Chase HP. Understanding insulin pumps and continuous glucose monitors. Denver (CO): Children's Diabetes Foundation; 2007.
14. McGarraugh G. The chemistry of commercial continuous glucose monitors. Diabetes Tech Therapeut 2009;11:S17–24.
15. Lagarde WH, Barrows FP, Davenport ML, et al. Continuous subcutaneous glucose monitoring in children with type 1 diabetes mellitus: a single-blind, randomized, controlled trial. Pediatr Diabetes 2006;7:159–64.
16. Garg S, Zisser H, Schwartz S, et al. Improvement in glycemic excursions with a transcutaneous, real-time continuous glucose sensor. Diabetes Care 2006;29:44–50.
17. Diabetes Research in Children Network (DirecNet) Study Group. Continuous glucose monitoring in children with type 1 diabetes. J Pediatr 2007;151:388–93.

18. Halvorson M, Carpenter S, Kaiserman K, et al. A pilot trial in pediatrics with the sensor-augmented pump: combining real-time continuous glucose monitoring with the insulin pump. J Pediatr 2007;150:103–5.
19. Schaepelynck-Belicar P, Vague P, Simonin G, et al. Improved metabolic control in diabetic adolescents using the Continuous Glucose Monitoring System (CGMS). Diabetes Metab 2003;29:608–12.
20. Ludvigsson J, Hanas R. Continuous subcutaneous glucose monitoring improved metabolic control in pediatric patients with type 1 diabetes: a controlled crossover study. Pediatrics 2003;111:933–8.
21. Juvenile Diabetes Research Foundation Continuous Glucose Monitoring Study Group—JDRF-CGM. The effects of continuous glucose monitoring in well-controlled type 1 diabetes. Diabetes Care 2009;32:1378–83.
22. Wolpert HA. Use of continuous glucose monitoring in the detection and prevention of hypoglycemia. J Diabetes Sci Technol 2007;1:146–50.
23. Wiltshire EJ, Newton K, McTavish L. Unrecognized hypoglycemia in children and adolescents with type 1 diabetes using the continuous glucose monitoring system: prevalence and contributors. J Paediatr Child Health 2006;42:758–63.
24. Gandrud LM, Xing D, Kollman C, et al. The Medtronic MiniMed Gold Continuous Glucose Monitoring System: an effective means to discover hypo- and hyperglycemia in children under 7 years of age. Diabetes Technol Ther 2007;9(4):307–16.
25. Schiaffini R, Ciampalini P, Fierabracii A, et al. The continuous glucose monitoring system (CGMS) in type 1 diabetic children is the way to recognize hypoglycemic risk. Diabetes/Metabol Res Rev 2002;18:324–9.
26. Tanenberg R, Bode B, Lane W, et al. Use of the continuous glucose monitoring system to guide therapy in patients with insulin-treated diabetes: a randomized controlled trial. Mayo Clin Proc 2004;79(12):1521–6.
27. Wadwa P, Fiallo-Scharer R, VanderWel B, et al. Continuous glucose monitoring in youth with type 1 diabetes. Diabetes Tech Therapeut 2009;11:S83–91.
28. Diabetes Research in Children Network (DirecNet) Study Group. Impact of exercise on overnight glycemic control in children with type 1 diabetes mellitus. J Pediatr 2005;147:528–34.
29. Hirsch IB, Abelseth J, Bode BW, et al. Sensor-augmented insulin pump therapy: Results of the first randomized treatment-to-target study. Diabetes Tech Therapeut 2008;10(5):377–83.
30. Deiss D, Bolinder J, Ribelin JP, et al. Improved glycemic control in poorly controlled patients with type 1 diabetes using real time continuous glucose monitoring. Diabetes Care 2006;29:2730–2.
31. Juvenile Diabetes Research Foundation Continuous Glucose Monitoring Study Group. Continuous glucose monitoring and intensive treatment of type 1 diabetes. N Engl J Med 2008;359:1464–76.
32. Juvenile Diabetes Research Foundation Continuous Glucose Monitoring Study Group—JDRF-CGM. Effectiveness of continuous glucose monitoring in a clinical care environment: evidence from the Juvenile Diabetes Research Foundation continuous glucose monitoring (JDRF-CGM) trial. Diabetes Care 2010;33(1):17–23.
33. Chase H, Beck R, Xing D, et al. Continuous glucose monitoring in youth with type 1 diabetes: 12-month follow-up of the Juvenile Diabetes Research Foundation continuous glucose monitoring trial. Diabetes Tech Therapeut 2010;12(7):507–15.
34. Cengiz E, Tamborlane W. A tale of two compartments: interstitial versus blood glucose monitoring. Diabetes Tech Therapeut 2009;11:S11–6.

35. Block J, Buckingham B. Use of real-time continuous glucose monitoring technology in children and adolescents. Diabetes Spectr 2008;21(2):84–90.
36. Messer L, Ruedy K, Xing D, et al. Education families on real time continuous glucose monitoring: the DirectNet Navigator Pilot Study Experience. Diabetes Educ 2009;35:124–35.
37. Wilson D. Impact of real-time continuous glucose monitoring on children and their families. J Diabetes Sci Technol 2007;1:142–5.
38. Gilliam L, Hirsch I. Practical aspects of real-time continuous glucose monitoring. Diabetes Tech Therapeut 2009;11:S75–82.
39. Block J. Continuous glucose monitoring: changing diabetes behavior in real time and retrospectively. J Diabetes Sci Technol 2008;2(3):484–9.
40. Blevins TC, Bode BW, Garg SK. Statement by the American Association of Clinical Endocrinologists Consensus Panel on Continuous Glucose Monitoring. Endocr Pract 2010;16(5):730–45.
41. Juvenile Diabetes Research Foundation Continuous Glucose Monitoring Study Group—JDRF-CGM. Factors predictive of use and of benefit from continuous glucose monitoring in type 1 diabetes. Diabetes Care 2009;32(11):1947–54.
42. Mackowiak L. Continuous glucose monitoring—getting started. Diabetes Self Manag 2007;24:15–20.
43. Edelman S, Bailey T. Continuous glucose monitoring health outcomes. Diabetes Tech Therapeut 2009;11:S68–74.
44. Diabetes Research in Children Network (DirecNet) Study Group. Use of the DirectNet Applied Treatment Algorithm (DATA) for diabetes management with a real-time continuous glucose monitor (the Freestyle Navigator). Pediatr Diabetes 2008;9:142–7.
45. Kowalski A. Can we really close the loop and how soon? Accelerating the availability of an artificial pancreas: a roadmap to better diabetes outcomes. Diabetes Tech Therapeut 2009;11:S113–9.
46. Brauker J. Continuous glucose sensing: future technology developments. Diabetes Tech Therapeut 2009;11(Suppl 1):S25–36.

Pain Management in the Pediatric Population

Lynn Clark, MS, RN, BC, CPNP-PC

KEYWORDS

- Pain • Pain management • Children • Opioid
- Nonsteroidal anti-inflammatory drugs
- Nonpharmacologic pain management

PAIN MANAGEMENT

Pain management is an important part of health care. There are very few encounters with health care providers that do not result in either physical or emotional pain. During childhood, the prevalence of pain depends on the child's ongoing health status. Most healthy children receive more than 20 immunizations before 2 years of age. If the child is born with health concerns and is required to spend time in the neonatal intensive care unit, the number of painful encounters can reach into the hundreds.

DEFINITION OF PAIN

Infants and young children are prone to experiencing undertreated or untreated pain because they are unable to verbalize exactly what is hurting or how much they are hurting. Critically ill and intubated children and adolescents are also at risk because of their inability to easily communicate. However, the child's inability to communicate does not make the health care provider exempt from responsibility to assess and treat pain. In these patients, it must be assumed that pain is present when children have painful medical conditions and/or are subjected to procedures that are painful.[1]

There are other well-accepted definitions of pain that have been around for many decades. Pain is subjective, therefore a clinician's ability to correctly estimate the amount of pain a patient is experiencing is highly inaccurate. McCaffery's definition states: "Pain is whatever the experiencing person says it is, and pain exists whenever the experiencing person says it does. Only the individual experiencing the pain is capable of truly describing its intensity, its nature, or its meaning. Thus, parents, physicians, and nurses can only guess at what a child is experiencing, and only the child can

Pain Management Department, Children's Medical Center Dallas, 1935 Medical District Drive, Dallas, TX 75235, USA
E-mail address: LYNN.CLARK@childrens.com

Crit Care Nurs Clin N Am 23 (2011) 291–301
doi:10.1016/j.ccell.2011.04.003
0899-5885/11/$ – see front matter © 2011 Elsevier Inc. All rights reserved.

give an accurate account of the experience."[2] Clinicians must obtain as much information from the child as possible to understand and decide what treatment method would best relieve the child's pain. Many factors influence the child's perception of pain, including past pain experiences, present coping skills, and parental anxiety and reaction. A child who has never been hospitalized and has never had surgery will have a different perspective on pain than a patient who has had a chronic, life-long illness requiring frequent health care visits. The child's subjective response is the best way to obtain information about his or her pain.

Pain is not merely a physiologic response to a noxious stimulus; emotions have a dramatic effect on pain. The International Association for the Study of Pain defines pain as "an unpleasant sensory and emotional experience associated with actual or potential tissue damage, or described in terms of such damage."[3(p210)] The child's (and family's) perception of pain produced by an emotional event, such as a traumatic injury, will be more intense than pain induced by a planned surgical intervention with expected outcomes.[4]

Fear and anxiety also have a large effect on pain in pediatric patients, which is especially true in procedural pain. A painful procedure, such as a dressing change, intravenous line placement, or even physical therapy sessions done with adequate pain control will influence the child's future response to pain. A procedure performed on a child with poor pain control will produce increased fear and anxiety, and will be apparent before the next painful procedure is begun. Care must be taken to provide adequate analgesia especially with the first procedure, as this will highly influence future pain perception for the child.[5]

EVOLUTION OF PEDIATRIC PAIN MANAGEMENT

Knowledge about pain transmission and pain perception in neonates has been a subject of study for several decades. Many myths persist despite evidence that pain can be transmitted and perceived during fetal development. Anand and colleagues[6] reported that at between 20 and 24 weeks of gestational age, all neural components for transmission of a pain signal from the periphery to the brain are intact; the neural pathway between the brain stem and thalamus are completely myelinated by 30 weeks of gestational age, meaning that pain signals are not only present but transmitted quickly. By 30 weeks' gestation, the pain signal from the periphery to the cerebral cortex can be recognized and perceived as pain by the fetus, producing systemic physiologic changes.

Ongoing painful experiences in the neonate, infant, or child lead to physiologic changes in the body. It was once believed that neonates had no ability to remember pain; however, like older children and adults, the experience associated with a painful event influences long-term pain memory. The experience of ongoing intermittent pain from heel sticks has been shown to contribute to long-term physical effects such as hyperalgesia.[7] When pain is present regularly the body begins to rewire at a cellular, synaptic, and molecular level. This plasticity is highest during the late prenatal and neonatal periods,[6] so repetitive procedures performed during this time have a significant impact on a child's future pain perception.

The physiologic effects of acute pain that is short in duration and quickly controlled are limited, and those changes will return to baseline with little long-term effect. However, painful events that occur frequently or have an extended duration decrease the body's ability to return to baseline. The memory of that pain experience is imprinted on the brain and spinal cord,[8] and remodeling occurs, changing future perception of pain.

PREVALENCE OF PAIN

Research on the prevalence of pain in the pediatric hospital setting is limited, but continues to support the assumption that pain in children is underassessed and/or undertreated. In the emergency room (ER), the prevalence of pain complaints on presentation is high. Cordell and colleagues[9] identified that 52.2% of adult patients who present to the ER have a chief complaint of pain. Pain is often a common complaint on presentation to the health care provider; however, it often remains undertreated during hospitalization.

Taylor and colleagues[10] reported that 77% of patients had some pain during their admission, with 23% reporting moderate to severe pain. Of these 23%, only 30% received some form of analgesic medication. These investigators also reported that 27% of hospitalized patients had pain before admission to the hospital, indicating a level of chronic pain in the pediatric population.

Ellis and colleagues[11] interviewed 237 hospitalized children and found that 20% reported severe pain during the 24 = hour study. It was also found that 34% of children had no analgesics ordered. Of the 157 children who did have analgesics ordered, 69% received none. Seven children were recognized as having poorly controlled pain, that is, their diagnoses included appendectomy, motor vehicle accident, and cervical spine injury, with the most common analgesic given being acetaminophen.

Chronic pain in the pediatric population is growing. A recent review by Malleson and Clinch[12] described data on common chronic pain conditions. The review found that back pain was present in about 30% of the community pediatric population. The study also listed other pediatric populations, with reports of increasing frequencies of chronic nonmalignant pain including diagnoses of hypermobility syndrome, juvenile idiopathic arthritis, chronic recurrent multifocal osteomyelitis, and cerebral palsy.

PHYSIOLOGIC EFFECTS OF ACUTE PAIN

In the acute phase, pain affects many systems within the body and causes a change in the body's physiologic response.[13(pp331–3)] **Table 1** provides an overview of the effects of pain on the systems within the body. The body's initial physiologic response—increased heart rate and blood pressure, and diaphoresis—does not remain present for as long as pain is present. The body's natural response to being revved up is to calm down. Patients who have chronic pain will not continue to have the same ongoing physiologic response unless an acute pain stimulus is once again introduced. Therefore, vital signs are not a good physiologic indicator of pain. Vitals signs may be used as a part of the pain assessment, but should not be used to rule out pain.[14]

LONG-TERM CONSEQUENCES OF ACUTE PAIN: POTENTIAL FOR PROGRESSION TO CHRONIC PAIN

When acute pain occurs, whether from mechanical, chemical, or thermal stimuli, the body produces chemical mediators in the periphery that start the process of pain transmission. The transient activation of the peripheral nociceptive fibers sends a signal of pain through the dorsal horn of the spinal cord to the brain, where that pain signal is perceived. Once the pain signal is received, the brain tells the body to remove itself from the painful stimulus. When the painful stimulus is no longer present, the pain signal is no longer being sent and the pain subsides.

Pain that is uncontrolled perpetuates and sustains current to the peripheral nociceptive fibers. This ongoing signal leads to sustained activation of the peripheral

Table 1
Physiologic effects of acute pain in children

System	Physiologic Effects
Endocrine system	Stress from pain causes a release of hormones, including cortisol, antidiuretic hormone, adrenocorticotropic hormone, growth hormone, catecholamines, and glucagon. It can also increase epinephrine and norepinephrine and decrease insulin and testosterone production. This increase in stress hormones can lead to increased catabolism and water retention, and increased metabolic rate. This increase in metabolism alters carbohydrate, protein, and fat intake, and can lead to hypoglycemia, weight loss, tachycardia, fever, and death
Immune system	The stress that results from pain suppresses the immune response, increasing risk for infection and sepsis
Pulmonary system	Pain can make it difficult to breathe normally, causing decreased flow, decreased volume, and decreased cough, which can lead to retained secretions, atelectasis, pneumonia, and infection. There may be decreased tidal volumes and lower vital lung capacity
Cardiovascular system	When pain occurs, the cardiovascular output increases. Pain causes increased heart rate, increased cardiac output, and increased systemic, peripheral, and coronary vascular resistance, leading to hypertension and increased myocardial oxygen consumption. Hypercoagulation and increased risk for deep vein thrombosis may also be present
Gastrointestinal system	Pain causes an increase in sympathetic tone. This sympathetic change increases intestinal secretions and smooth muscle tone, and may delay the return of gastric and bowel function
Cognitive and emotional system	Pain increases anxiety, fear, and confusion. Uncontrolled acute pain may lead to a long-term chronic pain condition, suffering, and disability

Table prepared using information from.[13,14]

nociceptive fibers, shifting the signal in the dorsal horn to a sensitized mode. Ongoing pain leads to central nervous system neuroplasticity, essentially rewiring the body for the transmission of constant pain signals, leading to chronic pain.[8]

BARRIERS TO OPTIMAL PAIN MANAGEMENT IN PEDIATRIC PATIENTS

Many factors, both internal and external, influence the individual prescribing the pain medication and the individual administering the pain medication. The acknowledgment of barriers that affect the delivery of pain relief will advance the ability to deliver optimal pain management. Each professional must be aware of any attitude or belief, personal opinion, or barrier that may influence the delivery of optimal pain management.

PHYSICIANS

Assessment and treatment decisions made by the health care team affect the adequacy of pain management. Pediatric patients are often inappropriately assessed and undermedicated, and consequently pain management is not optimal.[15–17] Physicians and other prescribing providers tend to order inadequate amounts, and occasionally inaccurate doses, of pain medications to be given only on an as-needed basis.[18]

The mismatch between the state of the science and the state of the practice has led to inadequate treatment of pain in pediatric patients. Pediatric residents have insufficient knowledge about how to assess pain and the use of pain medications in the patients they care for daily. Pediatric programs are required as per the guidelines of the Accreditation Council for Graduate Medical Education's (ACGME)[19] to ensure that residents can address pain associated with procedures and have "sufficient" training in pain management; however, they do not give specific requirements. Most surgical subspecialties, with the exception of neurosurgery and otolaryngology, have no requirement to teach their students about pain management.

Saroyan and colleagues conducted a study in 2008 that assessed resident knowledge of acute pain in hospitalized children. The investigators administered a questionnaire to anesthesia (25%), orthopedic (32%), and general pediatric (43%) residents. Although 85% of attending physicians and resident physicians rated the educational need for information about pediatric pain management to be moderate to high, pediatric residents, on average, answered fewer than 60% of the questions correctly. Most study participants (>70%) did not know that the Face, Legs, Activity, Cry, Consolability (FLACC) scale was appropriate for cognitively delayed patients, 70% did not know that the maximum daily dose of acetaminophen was 90 mg/kg/d, and fewer than 50% were able to use an equal analgesic chart to convert one opioid dosage to another. Education about pain management is lagging behind current and ever-evolving knowledge about pain management.[19]

NURSES

All health care providers, including nurses, can contribute to the problem of ineffective pain management. Nurses do not consistently assess infants and children with developmentally appropriate, valid, and reliable pain intensity scales.[20] Research indicates that nurses consistently rate patients' pain intensity lower than self-reports. Documentation of pain assessment is often infrequent and inconsistent. Communication between patient, family, nurse, and physician regarding pain may be incomplete and ineffective.[21–22] Nurses find that lack of valid pain assessment tools, poor documentation, and difficulty with pain assessment affects pain management for cognitively impaired pediatric patients.[23]

Nurses, empowered with analgesic prescriptions ordered as-needed, tend to undermedicate by administering dosages less often than prescribed.[17,18,20] Nurses also tend to choose the lowest opioid dosage or administer nonopioid analgesics instead of opioids. These choices may be based on inadequate or inappropriate knowledge, attitudes, and beliefs about pain assessment and pain management.[17,20]

ACHIEVING OPTIMAL PAIN RELIEF IN THE ACUTE CARE SETTING

When patients are experiencing acute pain, appropriate steps must be taken to optimize pain control to prevent long-term consequences. Adequate interventions cannot be initiated without first completing a thorough assessment of the patient. The clinician's ability to assess the patient's pain can be limited, due to the patient's age or developmental level and his or her inability to speak, as well as the patient being intubated and/or being sedated. Clinicians must use a valid, reliable, developmentally appropriate pain assessment scale to assist with their pain assessment. However, a pain intensity score is only one aspect of the assessment. Multidimensional tools are available that provide more information than a one-dimensional pain score, but there is no one convenient tool to provide a complete and comprehensive assessment of pain.

To provide optimal pain relief, it is necessary to continue to assess and reassess the patient's pain on a regular basis. The child who reports severe pain, receives an intervention, that is, medication or nonpharmacologic, and then is not reassessed until the next report of pain may never achieve ongoing relief. There is no confirmation that the dose of medication administered to the child provides adequate analgesia for the expected time or that the intervention is effective enough to decrease the child's pain. Reassessment after providing an intervention allows the provider to evaluate whether the intervention has been effective in relieving the child's pain. Pain scores are frequently used for reassessment, but the child's functionality should also be included. A normally active 4-year-old who reports that he or she is not hurting, but lies still in bed, may be experiencing more pain than he or she is reporting, and deserves further assessment and intervention.

When sudden, severe pain occurs in the acute care setting, there is an arsenal of medications available to treat the pain. Intravenous medications have a rapid onset, providing quick relief; however, the duration of relief is relatively short. Using only short-acting intravenous medications to treat pain creates many peaks and troughs in pain control. Pain occurs, intravenous medication is administered with rapid onset and short duration of relief, followed by a return of pain, and the cycle repeats. Oral medications take longer to be effective, but the duration of analgesia is longer. Using oral medications on a regular basis (when the child can tolerate oral medication) allows for a more consistent level of analgesia. The optimal pain medication regimen for short-term, acute pain (such as postsurgical pain) would include a medication that provided consistent relief (eg, consistently dosed short-acting oral pain medication, controlled-release oral medication, or an infusion of intravenous medication) with additional medication for breakthrough or severe pain (eg, short-acting oral or intravenous medication).

ALTERNATIVES FOR PAIN CONTROL

There also may be other options for pain control aside from medication. In a hospitalized patient with very complex medical problems, the first instinct is often to use medication as first-line intervention for pain control. Depending on the situation, this may be the correct decision; however, often some basic interventions remain untried. It should not be assumed that the most obvious cause for pain remains the patient's biggest irritation. Adjusting the patient in bed, providing ice or heat, or massage may decrease feelings of discomfort, while the medication relieves the pain. Using nonpharmacologic interventions in addition to medications is often necessary to optimize pain relief. Physical therapy and psychological support play an integral part in returning or maintaining function in children whose acute illness episode becomes extended.

Other options for pain control include interventional therapies such as epidural infusion, peripheral nerve infusion, nerve block, and continuous-infusion local anesthetic via preplaced catheters. The ability to use these options varies based on injury, chronic illness, infection, congenital abnormities, clotting ability, and a host of other factors. The use of interventional therapies can be helpful in reducing the amount of systemic opioids required to keep a child's pain adequately controlled.

In addition to acute pain due to injury or illness, hospitalized children often suffer pain from procedures. The prevention of procedure-related pain is an important aspect of pediatric pain management. Pediatric patients who must undergo bone marrow aspirates, lumbar punctures, fracture setting, chest tube placement, circumcision, or peripheral intravenous line insertion should be provided appropriate and adequate interventions to achieve optimal pain and anxiety control. There are many topical anesthetic options for patients requiring peripheral intravenous line placement; however, more invasive procedures may require sedation. The painfulness of the procedure and an evaluation of the child's ability to cope with the procedure are just two of the factors that should influence the decision about the most appropriate pain management intervention.

There is a multitude of pain medications available in many concentrations and routes, some more commonly used than others. In many instances, providers are knowledgable about a few medications and prescribe them frequently. When these common medications do not provide adequate relief, providers may lack knowledge about other options to change the regimen. Adequate pharmacologic and nonpharmacologic treatments exist to completely relieve pain. Changing to a multimodal pain management plan including adjuvants, nonpharmacologic modalities, and interventional pain management therapies in addition to changing the pain medication will have more favorable results than using just one modality.

TREATMENT THERAPIES

The cause of pain varies based on the injury or illness, and the perception of pain varies based on the patient. Acute pain of nociceptive origin can be treated with opioids and nonopioids, and nonpharmacologic interventions, with adequate outcomes. If acute pain remains untreated or undertreated and becomes chronic, it is much more difficult to treat and often takes a multimodal approach to provide relief and maintain function.

Pain management options include the following.

Nonopioids are used for mild to moderate pain or in addition to opioids for severe pain. The mechanism of action of acetaminophen is unknown, but there is evidence for central and peripheral nervous system effects. The maximum daily dose varies by age (90 mg/kg for children, 80 mg/kg for infants, 60 mg/kg for term neonates, and 45 mg/kg for preterm neonates).

Nonsteroidal anti-inflammatory drugs (NSAIDs). There are many NSAIDS available both by prescription and over the counter. The only NSAID available intravenously and orally is ketorolac. The most commonly used over-the-counter NSAID is ibuprofen, which is available for both oral and rectal routes. The use of NSAIDs may reduce overall opioid requirements. Caution should be exercised for patients with renal compromise and bleeding disorders, as NSAIDs may contribute to coagulopathy and increased blood loss.

Combination medications. These medications consist of an opioid combined with a nonopioid such as acetaminophen or ibuprofen. The dosing is limited to the amount of nonopioid in the medication. This type of medication is used for moderate to severe pain. Hydrocodone combined with acetaminophen or ibuprofen is the most commonly prescribed opioid. Acetaminophen with codeine has limited effectiveness in 5% to 10% of the Caucasian population and in 1% to 3% of African Americans who inherit low levels of enzyme used to metabolize the medication. More effective analgesics with fewer adverse effects have been developed, decreasing the use of acetaminophen with codeine in the pediatric population.

Opioids. Opioids are the natural, semisynthetic, and synthetic drugs that relieve pain by binding to opioid receptors in the body. Opioid is the preferred descriptor over narcotic, as the word narcotic has a very negative connotation in the community.[24] Oxycodone is available only in the oral formulation, but does have a controlled-release formulation. Hydromorphone is a potent analgesic that has few metabolites and is available in both oral and intravenous formulations. Morphine is considered the "gold standard," and is the most commonly used opioid. It does have active metabolites, namely, morphine-6-glucuronide, which is 2 to 25 times more potent as an analgesic than morphine, and morphine-3-glucuronide, which is inactive as an analgesic but may contribute to neurostimulatory effects and lead to toxicity if not excreted. Morphine has central effects within the spinal cord, including analgesia, respiratory depression, nausea and vomiting, miosis, increased prolactin release and general pituitary dysfunction, cough suppression and myoclonic muscle movements, tremor, and possible seizures at very high doses. Peripheral effects of morphine include histamine release, hypotension, increased gastrointestinal resting tone, decreased gastrointestinal propulsive movement, decreased biliary, intestinal, and pancreatic secretions, and immunosuppression. Meperidine should be reserved for very brief courses of administration in patients who have a demonstrated allergy or intolerance to other opioids. Meperidine has a toxic metabolite, normeperidine, which is a cerebral irritant, and accumulation can lead to seizures in otherwise healthy persons. Methadone is a unique synthetic long-acting opioid that may be effective for nociceptive and neuropathic pain. Methadone relieves pain by blocking N-methyl-D-aspartate glutamate receptors and µ receptors, and has a selective serotonin reuptake inhibitor (SSRI) mechanism. Patients who receive methadone long term develop less tolerance compared with other opioids. Methadone has no known active metabolites and is almost completely excreted in feces, therefore making it frequently used in patients with chronic renal failure. Methadone has the longest half-life of any opioid and therefore must be used with extreme caution, as the effects "stack" with repeated dosing, often requiring 48 to 72 hours to reach a steady-state blood level. There are many versions of conversion charts that suggest reasonable transition from morphine or other opioids to methadone. Conversion to methadone must be done cautiously (start low and titrate slowly) and the patient must be monitored for adverse effects, as the long half-life and stacking quality can result in delayed respiratory depression up to 72 hours after starting or increasing the dose.

Adjuvants. Drugs used to treat neuropathic pain generally target different receptors than do opioids. Anticonvulsants and tricyclic antidepressants were originally developed to treat conditions other than pain. Anticonvulsants, such as gabapentin, pregabalin, carbamazepine, and topiramate, affect neuronal firing by blocking sodium channels. Tricyclic antidepressants (TCAs), for example, amitriptyline and SSRIs such as cialopram, escitalorpam, and fluoxetine, inhibit the reuptake of serotonin and/or norepinephrine.

Other adjuvants such as muscle relaxants and benzodiazepines are used to treat conditions other than pain. Muscle relaxants, for example, baclofen, carisoprodol, methocarbamol, and tixanidine, are used to treat muscle spasms and relax tension that may be causing pain. Benzodiazepines, such as diazepam, lorazepam, and clonazepam, can be used to decrease spasm and/or anxiety, but benzodiazepines do not treat pain.

There are many other adjuvant medications in the arsenal of treatment modalities that can be used alone, but often in addition to other interventions. A multimodal approach is often the best way to optimize an individual plan for the patient. The term multimodal should not be confused with polypharmacy. Polypharmacy is the use of many drugs from the same class of medications. Multimodal is the use of multiple types of medications from varying classes and interventions, for example, opioids, nonopioids, TCAs, and nonpharmacologic methods, to fight pain at a variety of levels of the pain continuum.

Nonpharmacologic interventions should be used in addition to medications for acute pain, and can be more central for children with chronic pain. The method chosen for the child should be developmentally appropriate. Having the parents present can be beneficial, with appropriate instruction to guide them in their role. Parents may not have past experience to draw upon, so it is important to help them learn strategies that will assist the child with decreasing stress rather than magnifying pain perception. Infants and toddlers may find rocking and swaddling beneficial. Additional methods that can be taught and reinforced to the child during a stressful or painful experience include relaxation, distraction, guided imagery, biofeedback, and hypnosis. Physical methods, such as massage, the application of heat and cold, and transcutaneous electrical nerve stimulation cause the body to send signals other than pain through the nervous system.[25]

It is the responsibility of the health care provider to ensure that the child does not suffer from untreated pain or from pain inflicted during procedures. Many products exist to help reduce the pain from needle procedures. Some topical applications take only minutes to be effective, for example, jet-injected lidocaine/J-tip; other patches and creams, such as EMLA, LMX-4, and Synera, can take 30 to 60 minutes to be effective. Oral sucrose can be administered by pacifier or syringe as an option for procedural pain in the neonatal population. The decision about product selection should be based on the length of time available until the procedure is to be performed, the type of procedure, the child's age, and child/parent preference. As stated earlier, frequent painful procedures can lead to ongoing pain and a painful health care experience that the child will never forget.

When treating chronic pain in an acute care setting, it may be necessary to change the focus of the outcome. The goal of acute pain management is relief of pain caused by an acute illness or injury, whereas the goal of chronic pain management is to increase function and decrease suffering. The child may function daily with a constant amount of pain, so attempting to completely alleviate the child's chronic pain will be futile and unsuccessful. If the child with chronic pain becomes ill with an acute injury or illness, the goal becomes a return to baseline function and score.

NURSING CONSIDERATIONS

To optimally treat children with pain, nurses must realize that appropriately assessing and treating pain in children is a necessary part of their care. Pain that remains unassessed leads to untreated pain and ongoing suffering. Untreated or undertreated pain can lead to long-term chronic pain. Pain can remain undertreated because providers may have limited knowledge about options that affect assessment and treatment decisions. Health care professionals must take the time to equip themselves with current knowledge about pain assessment and treatment, and must also recognize that attitudes, beliefs, and previous experiences affect judgment. Pain is a subjective experience, and every child must be treated as an individual. Using a multimodal approach is the best way to optimize pain control, with the fewest adverse effects. Even the smallest child deserves the best pain control that can safely be achieved.

REFERENCES

1. Pasero C, McCaffery M. Pain in the critically ill: new information reveals that one of the simplest procedures—turning—can be the most painful one. Am J Nurs 2002; 102(1):59–60.
2. McCaffery M. Nursing practice theories related to cognition, bodily pain, and man-environment interactions. Los Angeles (CA): University of California at Los Angeles' Students' book store; 1968.
3. Merskey H, Bogduk N, editors. Classification of chronic pain. 2nd edition. Seattle (WA): IASP press; 1994.
4. Roy M, Piche M, Chen J, et al. Cerebral and spinal modulation of pain by emotions. Proc Natl Acad Sci U S A 2009;106(49):20900–5.
5. Zempsky W, Schechter N. What's new in the management of pain in children. Pediatr Rev 2003;24(10):337–47.
6. Anand S, Phil D, Hickey P. Pain and its effect in the human neonate and fetus. N Engl J Med 1987;317(21):1321–9.
7. Hermann C, Hohmeister J, Demirakc S, et al. Long-term alteration of pain sensitivity in school-aged children with early pain experiences. Pain 2006;125(3):278–85.
8. Carr D, Goudas L. Acute pain. Lancet 1999;353:2051–8.
9. Cordell W, Keene K, Giles B, et al. The high prevalence of pain emergency medical care. Am J Emerg Med 2002;20(3):165–9.
10. Taylor E, Boyer K, Campbell F. Pain in hospitalized children: a prospective cross-sectional survey of pain prevalence, intensity, assessment & management in a Canadian pediatric teaching hospital. Pain Res Manag 2008;13(1):25–32.
11. Ellis J, O'Connor B, Cappelli M, et al. Pain in hospitalized pediatric patients: how are we doing? Clin J Pain 2002;18:262–9.
12. Malleson P, Clinch J. Pain syndromes in children. Curr Opin Rheumatol 2003;15: 572–80.
13. Ecketerowicz N, Quinlan-colwell A, Vanderveer B, et al. Acute pain management. In: St Marie B, editor. Core curriculum for pain management nursing. 2nd edition. Philadelphia (PA): Saunders; 2010. p. 329–79.
14. McCaffery M, Herr K, Pasero C. Assessment tools. In: Pasero C, McCaffery C, editors. Pain assessment and pharmacologic management. St Louis (MO): Mosby; 2010. p. 49–142.
15. American Academy of Pediatrics, American Pain Society. The assessment and management of acute pain in infants, children and adolescents. Pediatrics 2001;108(3):793–7.
16. Cheng S, Foster R, Hester N. A review of factors predicting children's pain experiences. Issues Compr Pediatr Nurs 2003;26(4):203–16.
17. Vincent C, Denyes M. Relieving children's pain: nurses' abilities and analgesic administration practices. J Pediatr Nurs 2004;19(1):40–50.

18. Hamers J, Abu-Saad H, Van Den Hout M, et al. Are children given insufficient pain-relieving medication postoperatively? J Adv Nurs 1998;27(1):37–44.
19. Saroyan J, Schechter W, Tresgallo M, et al. Assessing resident knowledge of acute pain management in hospitalized children: a pilot study. J Pain Symptom Manage 2008;36(6):628–38.
20. Broome M, Huth M. Nursing management of the child in pain. In: Schechter N, Berde B, Yaster M, editors. Pain in infants, children and adolescents. 2nd edition. Philadelphia: Lippincott Williams & Wilkins; 2003. p. 417–33.
21. Griffie J. Addressing inadequate pain relief: effective communication among the health care team is essential. Am J Nurs 2003;103(8):61–3.
22. Van Niekerk LM, Martin F. The impact of the nurse-physician relationship on barriers encountered by nurses during pain management. Pain Manag Nurs 2003;4(1):3–10.
23. Malviya S, Voepel-Lewis T, Merkel S, et al. Difficult pain assessment and lack of clinical knowledge are ongoing barriers to effective pain management in children with cognitive impairment. Acute Pain 2005;7:27–32.
24. Pasero C, Quinn T, Portenoy R, et al. Opioid analgesics. In: Pasero C, McCaffery C, editors. Pain assessment and pharmacologic management. St Louis (MO): Mosby; 2010. p. 277–300.
25. DiMaggio T, Clark L, Czarnecki M. Pediatric pain management. In: St Marie B, editor. Core curriculum for pain management nursing. 2nd edition. Philadelphia (PA): Saunders; 2010. p. 481–542.

The 2010 American Heart Association Guidelines for Cardiopulmonary Resuscitation and Emergency Cardiac Care: An Overview of the Changes to Pediatric Basic and Advanced Life Support

Becky Spencer, MSN, RN[a,b,]*, Jisha Chacko, MS, RN[c],
Donna Sallee, MS, RN, FNP-C[a]

KEYWORDS

- Cardiopulmonary resuscitation • Pediatric basic life support
- Pediatric advanced life support • Infants • Children
- Defibrillation • Emergency cardiac care

The year 2010 celebrates the 50th anniversary of the development of cardiopulmonary resuscitation (CPR).[1] The American Heart Association (AHA) has a strong commitment to implementing scientific research–based interventions for CPR and emergency cardiovascular care (ECC). In 1992, the International Liaison Committee on Resuscitation (ILCOR) was created to bring together cardiopulmonary scientists

The authors have nothing to disclose.
[a] College of Nursing, Texas Woman's University, PO Box 425498, Denton, TX 76204, USA
[b] University of Kansas, School of Nursing, Kansas City, KS, USA
[c] 1261 McMahan Drive, Lewisville, TX 75077, USA
* Corresponding author. College of Nursing, Texas Woman's University, PO Box 425498, Denton, TX 76204.
E-mail address: bspencer@twu.edu

Crit Care Nurs Clin N Am 23 (2011) 303–310
doi:10.1016/j.ccell.2011.04.002
0899-5885/11/$ – see front matter © 2011 Published by Elsevier Inc.

ccnursing.theclinics.com

and experts from around the world to examine current research and formulate treatment recommendations.[2] This committee's work resulted in modifications to the AHA guidelines for CPR and ECC in 2000, 2005, and 2010. The 2010 AHA guidelines for CPR and ECC represent the consensus and culmination of the work of more than 350 resuscitation experts from 29 countries who reviewed thousands of studies and produced 411 scientific evidence reviews.[3] This article presents the 2010 AHA major guideline changes to pediatric basic life support (BLS) and pediatric advanced life support (PALS) and the rationale for the changes. The following topics are covered in this article: (1) current understanding of cardiac arrest in the pediatric population, (2) major changes in pediatric BLS, and (3) major changes in PALS.

CARDIAC ARREST IN THE PEDIATRIC POPULATION

The incidence of out-of-hospital pediatric cardiac arrest varies between 2 to 20 cases annually per 100,000 children.[4] Suominen and colleagues[5] report the in-hospital pediatric cardiac arrest incidence as 1% of all hospital admissions and 5.5% of pediatric intensive care unit admissions. Most episodes of cardiac arrest in children are caused by asphyxia.[6,7] Only 6.7% of all children who have an out-of-hospital cardiac arrest survive, and many of those who survive are neurologically impaired.[4] The survival rate of pediatric in-hospital cardiac arrest is approximately 27% to 30%.[8]

Factors that influence survival outcomes in patients with cardiac arrest include the environment in which the arrest occurs, the preexisting condition of the child, the length of time between the arrest and the initiation of CPR, the initial electrocardiographic rhythm detected, and the quality of the BLS and advanced life support interventions provided.[9] Many out-of-hospital cardiac arrests are not witnessed, and bystander CPR is initiated in only 30% of pediatric cardiac arrests.[10] Fast and effective bystander CPR is associated with successful return of spontaneous circulation (ROSC) as well as decreased neurologic sequelae.[11,12]

THE 2010 PEDIATRIC BLS GUIDELINES: MAJOR CHANGES
Age Range

According to the 2010 BLS guidelines, infant BLS guidelines only apply to infants younger than 1 year and child BLS guidelines apply to children approximately 1 year of age to puberty.[13] This is not a change for health care providers, but for lay rescuers; the child BLS guidelines were previously applied to children aged 1 to 8 years.[14] At present, the age guidelines for a child, 1 year to puberty, apply to all rescuers. For the purpose of CPR education, puberty is defined as breast development in adolescent girls and the presence of axillary hair in adolescent boys.[13]

Sequence

Change

The most notable difference in the 2010 guidelines is the change from the well-known sequence of A-B-C for airway, breathing, and circulation to C-A-B for circulation, airway, and breathing. If a pediatric patient is found unresponsive, or a witnessed cardiac arrest occurs, rescuers first provide 30 chest compressions, then open the airway, and then provide 2 rescue breaths.[15]

Rationale for change

The highest survival rates for cardiac arrest occur when the arrest is witnessed and the initial cardiac rhythm is ventricular fibrillation (VF) or pulseless ventricular tachycardia (VT).[2] VT and VF are not sustainable heart rhythms that deteriorate quickly to asystole without intervention. Beginning CPR with compressions supports circulatory perfusion during the critical time between the cardiac arrest and the acquisition of an automated external defibrillator (AED) or a manual defibrillator. Assar and colleagues[16] demonstrated that initiating CPR with 30 chest compressions followed by 2 ventilations leads to lesser delay in the initiation of compressions. Initiating CPR with 30 compressions would theoretically delay the ventilations by only 18 seconds or less.[15]

Some controversy exists in adopting C-A-B for pediatric patients with cardiac arrest. In infants and children, respiratory arrest is a more common cause of cardiac arrest than VF or VT. Ventilation is extremely important to a successful outcome in pediatric patients with cardiac arrest.[13] Kitamura and colleagues[12] found that resuscitation outcomes for respiratory arrest are better when ventilations and chest compressions are combined; however, the use of the C-A-B sequence was adopted for infants and children to simplify training, to provide consistency in training rescuers, and in the hope that more bystanders would provide early, high-quality CPR.[13]

Change
"Look, listen, and feel" after opening the airway to assess for presence of breathing was removed from the CPR sequence.

Rationale for change
The time taken to assess for breathing causes an additional delay and interruption in the circulatory perfusion provided by chest compressions.[15] Opening the airway and immediately giving 2 breaths as the second step of C-A-B minimizes the delay and interruption of chest compressions.

Change
An additional change to pediatric BLS guidelines is deemphasis of the pulse check. Lay providers do not check for a pulse as part of the CPR. The 2010 guidelines recommend that health care providers should attempt to check for a pulse for no longer than 10 seconds. "If, within 10 seconds, you don't feel a pulse or are not sure if you feel a pulse, begin chest compressions."[15]

Rationale for change
Evidence suggests that health care providers cannot reliably or rapidly detect the presence or absence of a pulse in children in emergency situations.[2] The deemphasis of this step was recommended to minimize delay in beginning chest compressions. Considering the risk of not providing chest compressions for a patient with cardiac arrest, the 2010 AHA guidelines recommend the provision of chest compressions if a rescuer is unsure about the presence of a pulse.[17]

Compression Depth

Change
Chest compressions in the pediatric patient should be at least one-third of the anterioposterior depth of the chest rather than one-third to half of the depth of the chest as designated by the AHA 2005 CPR guidelines.[14] This is approximately 1.5 in in infants and 2 in in children.[15]

Rationale for change
This change was made based on evidence obtained from radiologic studies, which determined that compressions of half the diameter of the anteroposterior chest wall may not be achievable.[15] Compressing one-third of the diameter of the chest provides adequate perfusion in an infant or a child.

Defibrillation and AED Use

Change
Defibrillation of infants with cardiac arrest is recommended. A manual defibrillator is preferred, but an AED with a pediatric dose attenuator can be used. If neither a manual defibrillator nor a pediatric dose attenuator is available, adult AED pads may be used.[15]

Rationale for change
"Although the safety of AEDs in infants <1 year of age is unknown, case reports have documented successful defibrillations in infants."[2] The current recommendation for energy dose for pediatric defibrillation is 2 to 4 J/kg delivered in a single shock.[2] Despite the lack of safety data, AED use in infants is recommended over no defibrillation at all.

THE 2010 PALS GUIDELINES: MAJOR CHANGES

In addition to the changes in the 2010 pediatric BLS guidelines, the PALS guidelines have also undergone some changes and refinement as a result of ILCOR's extensive literature review. The PALS cardiac arrest algorithm is now organized to encourage 2 minutes of uninterrupted CPR in between additional interventions to optimize perfusion through chest compressions.[15]

Defibrillation Dose

Change
As discussed in the AHA pediatric BLS guideline changes, the initial energy dose for defibrillation should be 2 to 4 J/kg. The AHA's recommendation is to start with 2 J/kg, but if refractory VF is present, 4 J/kg is acceptable. Additional shocks should be at least 4 J/kg but should not exceed 10 J/kg.[15]

Rationale for change
"Limited evidence is available about effective or maximum energy doses for pediatric defibrillation, but some data suggest that higher doses may be safe and potentially more effective."[15] This modification allows for a wider range of energy doses for more refractory pediatric cardiac arrest cases.

Carbon Dioxide Monitoring

Change
Health care providers should monitor exhaled carbon dioxide (CO_2) using capnography or colorimetry, if available, during CPR to assist in monitoring the effectiveness of chest compressions. Capnography or colorimetry should also be used in pediatric patients with a perfusing cardiac rhythm to confirm endotracheal tube placement and during patient transport.[17]

Rationale for change
In adult and animal studies, partial pressure of CO_2, end-tidal (P_{ETCO_2}) less than 10 to 15 mm Hg indicates potential overventilation.[17] Awareness of the P_{ETCO_2} level during resuscitation helps providers focus on effective compressions while moderating ventilations. "An abrupt and sustained rise in P_{ETCO_2} may be observed just before clinical identification of return of spontaneous circulation (ROSC), so use of P_{ETCO_2} monitoring may reduce the need to interrupt chest compressions for a pulse check."[15] Use of capnography or colorimetry also provides a faster indication of possible endotracheal tube displacement than an arterial blood gas.[15]

Oxygenation

Change

After ROSC, arterial oxyhemoglobin saturation should be monitored and the fraction of inspired oxygen (FIO_2) should be titrated to maintain an oxyhemoglobin saturation greater than or equal to 94%. If the oxyhemoglobin level is 100%, FIO_2 should be weaned to maintain not less than 94% saturation.[17]

Rationale for change

Kilgannon and colleagues[18] found that hyperoxia after resuscitation was an independent predictor of in-hospital mortality. A 100% oxyhemoglobin saturation level corresponds to a wide range of actual PaO_2 levels (80–500 mm Hg).[15] Titrating FIO_2 levels to maintain oxyhemoglobin saturation between 94% and 100% may reduce postresuscitation mortality.

Diagnostics

Change

The presence of wide-complex tachycardia is determined if the QRS width is greater than 0.09 seconds, which represents an increase from the 2005 AHA guidelines of 0.08 seconds.[17]

Rationale for change

Surawicz and colleagues[19] reported prolonged QRS complexes in children younger than 4 years at greater than 0.09 seconds, and in children aged 4 to 16 years at greater than 0.1 second. The AHA changed this determination to concur with these scientific recommendations.

Pharmacology

Change

Routine calcium administration is not recommended in pediatric cardiac arrest. Calcium may be considered for patients with documented hypocalcaemia, calcium channel blocker overdose, hypermagnesemia, or hyperkalemia.[15]

Rationale for change

Multiple studies reviewed by the ILCOR suggested a higher postresuscitation mortality rate in pediatric patients with cardiac arrest who received calcium during resuscitation.[17]

Change

Etomidate is a rapid acting hypnotic drug used as an anesthetic for endotracheal intubation.[20] The 2010 AHA guidelines advise against using etomidate in pediatric patients with evidence of septic shock.[17]

Rationale for change

Etomidate is associated with decreased cortisol plasma levels. Studies of etomidate use in adults and children indicate higher mortality rates among patients with septic shock possibly related to the inhibitory effects on corticosteroid synthesis.[17]

Special Considerations

Change

Extracorporeal cardiac life support (ECLS) is an acceptable consideration for infants and children with congenital heart anomalies including single-ventricle anatomy and Fontan or hemi-Fontan/bidirectional Glenn physiology.[17] ECLS may also be considered in pediatric patients with cardiac arrest with pulmonary hypertension or environmentally induced severe hypothermia.[17]

Rationale for change
Studies regarding the use of ECLS show mixed results. The present ILCOR consensus supports the potential use of ECLS in pediatric patients with cardiac arrest having an underlying cardiac condition or severe hypothermia but reject the use of ECLS in pediatric patients with cardiac arrest with no underlying cardiac disease.[17]

Change
"Therapeutic hypothermia (32°C to 34°C) may be beneficial for adolescents who remain comatose after resuscitation from sudden witnessed out-of-hospital VF cardiac arrest."[15] Infants and children who remain comatose after resuscitation may also be considered for therapeutic hypothermia.

Rationale for change
Research investigating induced therapeutic hypothermia up to 72 hours after resuscitation in adults with VF arrest and infants with birth asphyxia demonstrated an acceptable safety profile and a possible association with better long-term neurologic outcomes.[17]

Change
All infants, children, adolescents, and young adults should have an "unrestricted complete autopsy, preferably performed by a pathologist with training and expertise in cardiovascular pathology."[15] A complete medical and family history should also be obtained. Genetic analysis for channelopathic causes for sudden death on tissue samples should also be completed.

Rationale for change
Channelopathies are inherited abnormalities of myocardial ion channels that can cause fatal arrhythmias.[17] Genetic testing and counseling for living family members of affected persons is vital for the identification and treatment of those at risk for sudden cardiac death in families.

Change
When possible, family members should be allowed to be with their child during in-hospital resuscitation.[17]

Rationale for change
Several researchers indicated that family members want to have the option of being present during resuscitation of their children and thought that their presence was beneficial to the child.[17] Additional studies revealed that family presence during in-hospital resuscitation did not negatively affect health care staff or their abilities to perform resuscitation.[17]

Nursing Implications
The 2010 AHA guidelines for CPR and ECC are the result of a tremendous effort to implement scientific evidence directly to patient care with the goal of improving clinical outcomes after resuscitation. The AHA continues to place emphasis on early and effective compressions, and early defibrillation, because these interventions consistently increase survival rates after cardiac arrest as evidenced in the literature. All nurses have a responsibility to be adequately trained in CPR and to implement evidence-based practice into their care. Nurses have a vast scope of practice in which knowledge and comfort with BLS and ECC skills are critically important. Nurses

represent one profession in a multidisciplinary health care team when responding to cardiac arrest situations. The 2010 AHA CPR and ECC guidelines also place greater emphasis on "team resuscitation," noting that BLS health care training should focus on teaching rescuers to work effectively in teams.[15] Mock codes in hospitals should encourage collaboration among health care providers in delegation of tasks and seamless coordination of different roles assumed, such as compressions, ventilations, medication administration, recording, and defibrillation, in an effort to provide efficient and effective resuscitations. As trusted members of communities, nurses also have a great opportunity to share the 2010 AHA/ECC guideline changes and encourage patients, families, and members of our communities to learn CPR. The evidence strongly suggests that increased survival rates and improved clinical outcomes after cardiac arrest are possible for infants and children, as well as adults. Update your skills and spread the word.

REFERENCES

1. American Heart Association. History of cardiopulmonary resuscitation. Available at: http://www.heart.org/HEARTORG/CPRAndECC/WhatisCPR/CPRFactsandStats/History-of-CPR_UCM_307549_Article.jsp. Updated February, 8 2011. Accessed April 1, 2011.
2. Nolan JP, Hazinski MF, Billi JE, et al. Part 1: executive summary: 2010 International Consensus on Cardiopulmonary Resuscitation and Emergency Cardiovascular Care Science With Treatment Recommendations. Resuscitation 2010;81(Suppl 1):e1–25.
3. Nolan JP, Nadkarni VM, Billi JE, et al. Part 2: international collaboration in resuscitation science: 2010 International Consensus on Cardiopulmonary Resuscitation and Emergency Cardiovascular Care Science with Treatment Recommendations. Resuscitation 2010;81(Suppl 1):e26–31.
4. Donoghue AJ, Nadkarni V, Berg RA, et al. Out-of-hospital pediatric cardiac arrest: an epidemiologic review and assessment of current knowledge. Ann Emerg Med 2005;46(6):512–22.
5. Suominen P, Olkkola KT, Voipio V, et al. Utstein style reporting of in-hospital paediatric cardiopulmonary resuscitation. Resuscitation 2000;45(1):17–25.
6. Hickey RW, Cohen DM, Strausbaugh S, et al. Pediatric patients requiring CPR in the prehospital setting. Ann Emerg Med 1995;25(4):495–501.
7. Berg MD, Schexnayder SM, Chameides L, et al. Pediatric basic life support: 2010 American Heart Association Guidelines for Cardiopulmonary Resuscitation and Emergency Cardiovascular Care. Pediatrics 2010;126(5):e1345–60.
8. Nadkarni VM, Larkin GL, Peberdy MA, et al. First documented rhythm and clinical outcome from in-hospital cardiac arrest among children and adults. JAMA 2006; 295(1):50–7.
9. Topjian AA, Berg RA, Nadkarni VM. Pediatric cardiopulmonary resuscitation: advances in science, techniques, and outcomes. Pediatrics 2008;122(5):1086–98.
10. Young KD, Seidel JS. Pediatric cardiopulmonary resuscitation: a collective review. Ann Emerg Med 1999;33(2):195–205.
11. Hickey RF, Cason BA. Timing of tracheal extubation in adult cardiac surgery patients. J Card Surg 1995;10(4 Pt 1):340–8.
12. Kitamura T, Iwami T, Kawamura T, et al. Conventional and chest-compression-only cardiopulmonary resuscitation by bystanders for children who have out-of-hospital cardiac arrests: a prospective, nationwide, population-based cohort study. Lancet 2010;375(9723):1347–54.

13. Berg MD, Schexnayder SM, Chameides L, et al. Part 13: pediatric basic life support: 2010 American Heart Association Guidelines for Cardiopulmonary Resuscitation and Emergency Cardiovascular Care. Circulation 2010;122(18 Suppl 3): S862–75.

14. Hazinski MF, Nadkarni VM, Hickey RW, et al. Major changes in the 2005 AHA Guidelines for CPR and ECC: reaching the tipping point for change. Circulation 2005;112(Suppl 24):IV206–11.

15. Hazinski MF, Nolan JP, Billi JE, et al. Part 1: executive summary: 2010 International Consensus on Cardiopulmonary Resuscitation and Emergency Cardiovascular Care Science With Treatment Recommendations. Circulation 2010; 122(16 Suppl 2):S250–75.

16. Assar D, Chamberlain D, Colquhoun M, et al. Randomised controlled trials of staged teaching for basic life support. 1. Skill acquisition at bronze stage. Resuscitation 2000;45(1):7–15.

17. de Caen AR, Kleinman ME, Chameides L, et al. Part 10: paediatric basic and advanced life support: 2010 International Consensus on Cardiopulmonary Resuscitation and Emergency Cardiovascular Care Science with Treatment Recommendations. Resuscitation 2010;81(Suppl 1):e213–59.

18. Kilgannon JH, Jones AE, Shapiro NI, et al. Association between arterial hyperoxia following resuscitation from cardiac arrest and in-hospital mortality. JAMA 2010; 303(21):2165–71.

19. Surawicz B, Childers R, Deal BJ, et al. AHA/ACCF/HRS recommendations for the standardization and interpretation of the electrocardiogram: part III: intraventricular conduction disturbances: a scientific statement from the American Heart Association Electrocardiography and Arrhythmias Committee, Council on Clinical Cardiology; the American College of Cardiology Foundation; and the Heart Rhythm Society. Endorsed by the International Society for Computerized Electrocardiology. J Am Coll Cardiol 2009;53(11):976–81.

20. Drug Information Online. Etomidate. Available at: http://www.drugs.com/pro/etomidate.html. Updated July 1, 2011. Accessed April 1, 2011.

Young Adults with Risk Factors for Chronic Disease: Transition Needs for Survivors of Childhood Cancer

Lisa M. Bashore, PhD, RN, CPNP, CPON

KEYWORDS

• Transition • Chronic illness • Young adults • Survivorship
• Cancer

Almost 80% of the children diagnosed with cancer in the past 10 years will now become a 5-year survivor, and 1 in 570 individuals between the ages of 20 and 34 years is a survivor of childhood or adolescent cancer.[1] Survivors living well into adulthood may develop or be at significant risk for developing chronic diseases.[2] Institutions may vary on how they institute the transition of care for the pediatric cancer survivor who is now an adult requiring adult-focused survivorship care.[3] This article includes a definition of transition, the current state of transition, a review of transition research, an overview of chronic disease in survivors of childhood cancer (SCC), and the transition of SCC. In addition, models of transition are discussed, and the barriers to transition as well as principles for successful transition are identified.

WHAT IS TRANSITION

The word transition has been defined in many ways, and transition from a nursing perspective is a central concept for nursing.[4] Transition as used in the care of cancer survivors has been defined as the passage from one state or place to another.[5] Transition is not a linear movement from pediatric to adult care but a movement or change that often takes many different directions in response to life events.[6] For example, Kralik and colleagues[7(pxii)] proposed that transition is neither an event nor a change but an inner reorientation and self-redefinition that individuals go through in response

---

The author has nothing to disclose.
Life After Cancer Program, Cook Children's Medical Center, 7th Avenue, Suite 220, Fort Worth, TX 76104, USA
E-mail address: Lisa.bashore@cookchildrens.org

doi:10.1016/j.ccell.2011.02.002
0899-5885/11/$ – see front matter © 2011 Elsevier Inc. All rights reserved.
ccnursing.theclinics.com

to change like survivors who experience late complications of their cancer treatment. Transition is a psychological process in the adaptation to a disruption or change. For children, adolescents, and young adults (YAs) with cancer, changes occur during the movement from acute cancer therapy to survivorship. Transitions occur for cancer survivors from pediatric to adult care practitioners. In all instances, the results include psychological responses, including anxiety, uncertainty, and concern over unmet medical needs of survivors with chronic disease.

Transition has been defined and reviewed extensively in the literature because it relates to chronic illness for several diseases, including sickle cell disease, cystic fibrosis (CF), solid organ transplants, and cancer.[8–15] The purpose of this article is not to provide a critique or an extensive review of the literature regarding transition but to continue the discussion of transition of YAs to appropriate adult services for YA childhood cancer survivors (YACCS) with both identified chronic diseases and those at risk for the development of chronic illness. An extensive review of the literature of transition of adolescents specifically with special health care needs indicated that most of the research conducted evaluating transition programs lack sound theoretical frameworks, design, and lack of control groups to evaluate transition services for adolescents and YAs (AYAs) with special health care needs.[16]

Nurses can play a critical role in conducting studies regarding the transition of AYAs to adult services. Nurses are also responsible for the education of survivors and their families about the benefits of transition and can assist survivors, especially, to overcome the many obstacles to transition of care. Because of the vast number of developmental changes occurring during adolescence in particular, parents, nurses, and other health providers should begin the discussion of transition early. As adolescence becomes reality, it signifies a time of significant change and transformation in the lives of adolescents, and the introduction of transition to young adulthood is reasonable. Practitioners should be using the normal developmental processes occurring during this time, for example, formation of identity and autonomy as prime interludes in which to introduce the concept of transition, so it then becomes a natural part of the information shared with adolescents during clinic visits.

THE STATE OF TRANSITION

Unfortunately, in many institutions, there are no policies governing the transition of care for AYAs in general or for YAs with chronic disease. The editorial commentary reported the need for quality health care for AYAs with chronic diseases, including YACCS at risk for late effects of cancer therapy.[17] Sawyer[17] cited a comment by Dr T Cull in 2008, which suggested that the improved survival of chronic illnesses results in a tsunami of chronically ill YAs. The past and current state of health transitions for AYAs and changes within both pediatric and adult health care systems were evaluated to ascertain successful transitions for children to adult services.[18] The researchers recommended educating professionals about how to terminate care of a patient and how to work with other agencies and organizations to establish an environment for successful transition. Until such time, because formal standardized policies exist, transition and the barriers to transition will continue to impede the emergence of functional YAs. The same barriers to successful transition of older AYA cancer survivors exist for many pediatric oncology programs.

In 2002, the American Academy of Pediatrics, the American Academy of Family Physicians, the American College of Physicians, and the American Society of Internal Medicine and, in 2003, the Society for Adolescent Medicine published position statements on the transition of children, adolescents, and YAs with chronic disease and with specialized health care needs.[19,20] Unfortunately, not all of the public sector, including pediatricians, internists, and health care institutions, established formal policies for the successful transition of YAs with chronic illness (YACI) to appropriate care.

More recently in 2009, the Society for Adolescent Medicine published a position paper describing the effect of health care reform and adolescent health care.[21] Although this position paper does not specifically address the transition of AYAs with chronic disease, it does present the principles of YA as they related to health care. The principles of the health care reform and their rationale for adolescents are found in **Table 1**.

Nurses play an important role in initiating and supporting policies, which guide transition services for the YACI and play a vital role in the healthy and smooth transition of YAs. Transition needs to be included in the plan of care for any child diagnosed with a potentially chronic health condition.[22–25] Having an adult practitioner who can potentially manage all of the survivors' medical needs or a community model of survivor care may be the most realistic of models for survivor care. Institutional policies describing the transition process and setting the guidelines on whom and when they get transitioned to adult health care providers are necessary to make any transition program a success. Adolescents with chronic conditions also require special services through school, work, and home. Ascertaining that the adolescent with special health needs, such as survivors of cancer, are integrated into these services is an important role of the pediatric nurse and practitioner during the transition process.[26] Nurses can support the students'

Table 1	
Principles of transition	
Principle	**Rationale**
Health care needs of AYAs should be financially accessible	Efforts should be made to ensure that coverage for all youth is covered under health care reform. Specifically, coverage should be covered under federally funded programs
A comprehensive list of services should be available for adolescents with special needs	Health care coverage should be more comprehensive, covering a wide range of services, including preventative health care and mental health benefits
A wide range of health professionals trained to meet the health care needs of AYAs should be available	Education programs should address the specific health care needs of AYAs with special health care needs. Training programs should be developed to meet the health care needs of AYAs. Reimbursement for the services provided should also be included, as well as support for the AYA programs
Confidentiality of the adolescent's health care records must be maintained	Support the confidentiality of adolescents to encourage further development of independence in meeting their own health care needs
The needs of special groups of adolescents should be met	Many adolescents have special needs, but in those with chronic physical and mental health conditions, it is important to be sure that their coverage continues well into adulthood

Data from English A, Park MJ, Shafer MA, et al. Health care reform and adolescents-an agenda for the lifespan: a position paper of the society of adolescent medicine. J Adolesc Health 2009; 45(3):310–5.

academic and vocational success by making sure that they are suitably referred to the appropriate services, including the disability office in a college. Many YA survivors of cancer with chronic health conditions resulting from their treatment and other YACI may require disability benefits to be able to receive necessary medical services.

TRANSITION RESEARCH

Kirk[10] addressed the transition needs of several YAs with more complex health care needs. Many of the young individuals studied indicated a concern about being in limbo regarding where or who would they seek support from in the event they needed services. Others talked about the differences between pediatric services and adult services. Children's hospitals were viewed as warm, friendly, and protective, whereas the adult facilities were perceived as being more depersonalized and threatening to them. Despite the negativity of the adult services, many of these participants and YAs in Tuchman and colleagues'[14] and Kirk's[10] study reported that they are seen as an adult. The adult practitioners addressed their questions to them and encouraged the YA to be the decision maker. Participants reported that they liked and appreciated the idea of the adult provider asking them what they thought and that decisions were theirs to make. Healthy transition to adult care includes the support and focus on the older AYAs' emotional development during a critical phase during their lives. During this time, YAs are pursuing life goals and establishing their identities, and any disruptions in the pursuit of good health and goal achievement may result in reduced well-being.

The course of life was examined in a large population of Dutch YAs with several chronic illnesses, including anorectic malformations, Hirschsprung disease, esophageal atresia, end-stage renal disease, and childhood cancer.[12] The SCC had lower social development and had achieved fewer milestones, including autonomy as well as psychosexual and social development. The findings of this study are important to recognize for SCC in particular when initiating transition services. Because of the potentially life-threatening nature of cancer and the dependency on their parents as children with cancer, SCC often have less participation in school and other peer activities. The lack of a healthy normal childhood, peer relations, and social development could potentially threaten a successful transition to adult care. Adolescents with congenital heart disease (CHD) now live well into adulthood, and the transition of care for these emerging YAs has been studied for some time, yet little data exist on the best way to transition these YAs for ongoing follow-up care.[27] One of the limitations of the research on children with CHD is that those children who no longer receive services or who have yet to develop complications as a result of their CHD are not included. Like SCC, adult survivors of childhood CHD have unrealized chronic diseases as a result of their childhood illness and require ongoing surveillance as adults.[27]

The transition of care for YACI was recently examined using national survey data from both general internists and pediatricians.[28] The survey explored attitudes toward and barriers to continued care of YACI and identified many barriers to both care and transition of care for the YACI. The transition from general pediatric to adult care identified that one of the biggest barriers to transition to adult care was the inability of pediatricians to let go of their patients.[29] Internists also reported barriers to caring for these YAs with chronic diseases, including the lack of reimbursement for the care provided and their own lack of access to appropriate resources to manage YACI.[28]

CHRONIC DISEASE IN CANCER SURVIVORS

Chronic disease or health conditions can be defined as those disorders that have a biologic, cognitive, or psychological basis and have lasted or are expected to last for more than 1 year.[11] Further, these disorders are expected to result in one or more of the following outcomes:

1. Limitations of function or a social role when compared with healthy peers with respect to physical, emotional, cognitive, or social growth and development
2. A dependency on medications, diet, assistive devices, medical technology, or personal assistance to function or participate in social activities
3. A need for social, medical, psychological, or educational services more than what would be usual to accommodate for education, home, or vocational success.

The concept of chronic disease in SCC is also well described.[30–32] The Children's Cancer Survivors Study was a retrospective cohort study that tracked more than 14,000 long-term SCC treated from 1970 to 1986. Many of these survivors are now well into adulthood and are experiencing several realized chronic health conditions, including congestive heart failure, second malignant neoplasms,[31] stroke,[32] and cognitive dysfunction.[33] The development of any of these late complications of childhood cancer therapy may result in chronic health conditions for survivors.

Oeffinger and colleagues[2] reported on the self-reported chronic illness in survivors and revealed that the cumulative incidence of chronic disease was at least 66% 25 years after treatment, and there was an estimated incidence of chronic illness in survivors of 73% (95% CI, 69.0%–77.9%) at 30 years after completion of therapy.[2] Survivors in this study reported a grade 3 to 5 chronic disease. A grade 3 disability results in a severe disabling condition, whereas a grade 5 disability results in a fatal outcome. The cumulative incidence of developing a chronic disease at 25 years after diagnosis was 42.4% at 30 years. The onset of many of the chronic diseases in cancer survivors may begin in adolescence and progressively worsen as they get older.

Central nervous system (CNS) tumor survivors have an increased risk for developing chronic illness, including obesity and endocrine issues, predisposing them to other ill health effects.[34] Health concerns include growth and thyroid deficiencies that may cause poor bone health, abnormalities in lipid profile, and adrenal insufficiency.

Chronic disease in childhood and adolescence results in delays in development in all domains, including not only the physical domain but also the social and emotional domains.[35] The effects of these delays in development can result in problems with social networking and peer development. Further, many YAs with chronic disease may not "fit in" with peers of their same age because of developmental delays. Many AYAs with significant delays in social and cognitive development also have poorer school performance. The ability to effectively transition older AYAs with chronic disease is marred not only by the medical issues but also by the multiple social and emotional issues these YAs face as they age.

The health-related hindrance (HRH) and personal goal pursuit were explored in a population of YACCS and YAs with CF compared with YAs without chronic illness.[36] HRHs are health events that impair the success of YAs in being successful in achieving their personal career goals. YAs with late effects and reduced lung function for CF survivors were more likely to have HRHs. These findings indicated a need to address the potential effect of having identified health problems and their subsequent effect on the well-being and healthy pursuit of goals in YAs with chronic disease.

TRANSITION OF YACCS

Cancer is a chronic disease, and several adult SCC deal with indolent cancers or experience a secondary malignancy that may be best managed within a model that uses an interdisciplinary approach. However, the reality for many YA and adult SCC is the lack of access to adult services and, more importantly, multidisciplinary services. Because of the risk for potential chronic disease and concomitant chronic disease in these survivors, medical oncologists alone may not be sufficient to manage the myriad of issues these survivors face. Community physicians, such as internists, are able to manage the many potential chronic diseases that may occur in YACCS. However, the Creating Healthy Futures (CHF) transition program as proposed by Betz and Redcay[37,38] within the community setting may be the most successful model for YACCS with chronic illness. The CHF program uses transition service coordinators (TSCs) who are nurse practitioners whose roles include the following: expert, consultant, leader, researcher, and educator. The primary function of the TSC is to coordinate the transition process for adolescents.

YA cancer survivors benefit from transition to adult services for multiple reasons, including receiving the best and most appropriate medical follow-up by practitioners with expertise in adult care. SCC are at risk for and already have chronic health conditions because of cancer treatment. The late effects of therapy and the need for ongoing adult follow-up management cannot be underscored. Many adult providers are in the best position to provide evaluation and management of a vast number of chronic diseases. The transition of YACCS to the best available medical professional will serve several purposes. First, survivors with chronic disease will receive the most benefit from services directed by medical internists and other adult providers with expertise in chronic disease. Second, integrating the approach Betz and Redcay[23,37,38] developed within a community model for YACI as YACCS will assure that educational, vocational, and other support services are provided.

Pediatric oncology programs are not equipped to manage all of the health needs of cancer survivors. However, pediatric oncology programs are better equipped to educate, because of the expertise of staff in cancer survivorship, and also to prepare survivors for transition. Early communication between pediatric oncology survivor services and adult practitioners should begin in adolescence to avoid gaps in medical care and to allow ample time for all parties to become familiar with the medical and psychosocial concerns of the adolescent and/or YA.

MODELS OF TRANSITION

The transition of YACCS from a pediatric center to adult services is not a new concept. Models for survivorship care exist within survivor programs to adequately and formally evaluate and manage the potential chronic diseases in survivors and the concomitant chronic diseases in the survivors.[39] Several cancer survivor programs have formal, comprehensive, interdisciplinary transition programs to adult services. These programs exist to ascertain that the long-term health care needs of cancer survivors are met using a collaborative approach between the oncology center, primary care physicians, and adult practitioners in the community.[39] Advanced practice nurses (APNs) and coordinators are included in the programs to support the healthy transition of the YACCS. Current models of survivorship transition programs have had success both because of funding and the vast experience and expertise of the researchers and clinicians who have made it a success. Other collaborative programs exist across the country to meet the medical needs of the growing number of YACCS. Scal and colleagues[40] conducted a study examining 122 transition programs and the documented services each of them provided. The programs fell into 4 categories, including a disease-specific model, a subspecialty model, an adolescent health model, and a primary care model. None of the transition programs provided the comprehensive services the programs claimed were necessary for the healthy transition of adolescents to adult care. The reasons for the shortcomings of the transition programs already established are not clear and could be because of the lack of resources, such as money, staff, and the ability of personnel to follow-through on designed services.

The most important transitions are for those YA survivors most significantly affected by cancer therapy. Henderson and colleagues[3] proposed a risk-based focused survivor care model of care and described the need to ensure that the most impaired survivors as well as survivors at risk for developing late effects received appropriate survivor care. Survivors of CNS tumors are most likely to experience late complications of therapy because of the tumor location and the effect on multiple organ systems.[34] The endocrine, cardiovascular, neurologic, dental, sensory, and immune systems are all affected by the treatment of CNS tumors. Many survivors of CNS tumors are treated with CNS-directed radiation therapy irrespective of age, but the treatment has potentially devastating late complications.[34]

Eshelman-Kent and colleagues[34] pointed out the likely barriers to transition for this group of survivors and described the various models in which to transition this group of survivors. The concern for these YACCS is to be sure that their ongoing medical, social, and emotional needs are met. Further, the best model to address the late effects for CNS survivors should be chosen. Risk-based, focused care is ideal, but a question arises about who should be providing that care. The adult practitioner has limited knowledge in the vast number of late complications for SCC, and the pediatric center may not be equipped to manage the chronic diseases faced by these survivors.

BARRIERS TO TRANSITION

Multiple barriers to successful transition of YA to adult services exist and are similar to barriers faced by YACCS.[9,15,37] The barriers facing YACCS are similar to most programs and include the patient and their families, the providers, and the health care system and are summarized in **Table 2**. Barriers include pediatric providers and their mistrust of the ability of adult providers to provide best care. Other barriers include the patient and parents who have emotional ties to the pediatric health care system, fear of the unknown, and lack of maturity most likely because of the dependency on pediatric staff. Other barriers are the adult provider who is both busy and not educated on the vast number of needs that may be facing the YA survivor of childhood chronic disease and the lack of educational programs focusing on chronic disease in YACCS.[3,15,28,41]

Many pediatric oncologists continue to manage the medical needs of YACCS; therefore, a number of YACCS may not be receiving the most appropriate medical and support services necessary for healthy development as a YA. The YACCS remaining exclusively under the care of pediatric oncologists may never fulfill the need to become independent, autonomous, and functional YAs but rather continue to rely and depend on their parents and their pediatric health providers and staff to meet their needs.

AYA opinions serve as barriers to successful transition to adult care. The concerns about transition in 22 AYAs were examined in a recent study.[14] Over time, most AYAs indicated a trend toward positive attitudes about transition despite early negative opinions about having to transition to adult care. The timing of transition is an important concept to consider when transitioning any adolescent or YA with chronic illness. Transition, as previously defined, is a process, which evolves over time and is a reorientation to change. This study emphasized the need to include the active participation of the adolescent regarding what could potentially enhance their transition to adult care. The AYAs in this study by Tuchman and colleagues[14] indicated that they expected the clinical practice to which they would be transitioned to be fair and

Table 2
Barriers to transition of YACI and YACCS to adult services

Barriers to Transition	Issues
Patient	Dependency and immaturity Lack of trust Severity of illness
Survivor (YACCS)	Severity of illness Knowledge deficits about treatment No need for prevention Lack of access to health care
Family	Need for control Lack of trust Overprotection
Pediatric oncologist	Lack of trust in adult providers or pediatricians Emotional ties to patients and survivors Comfort in caring for YACI, including late effects in YACCS Lack of communication between providers
Adult providers	Knowledge deficits in late effects of cancer Knowledge deficits about chronic illness in children Lack of commitment Lack of specialized training
Health care system	Access issues (insurance, financial, availability) Few formal transition programs Lack of formal guidelines Lack of funding for research and transition programs for survivors

Data from Refs.[3,15,28,41]

consistent among all AYAs, which may be difficult because of the disease severity and cognition of many AYAs. Many participants indicated a positive experience once they were transitioned and could identify the benefits of being part of an adult center, including independence and responsibility for their own care as adults.

The health care environment is another barrier to transition of YACCS. Without adequate insurance, the accessibility of special health services programs may not be possible. English and colleagues[21] suggested that health care reforms provide for services, such as mental health services, substance abuse programs, and family planning programs, to be offered as government-supported programs. Services in these sectors should be available to YAs irrespective of health insurance coverage. Health care reform policies should begin to better reimburse for preventative health services for the chronically ill AYA.

SCC like others with childhood illnesses experience less social development and have not acquired many developmental milestones that hamper successful transition to adult services.[12] Cancer survivors should be encouraged to engage in independent behaviors in adolescence so that they can best cope with the challenges of adulthood. These survivors should be encouraged to participate in social activities with their peers and maintain the social contacts they made before and during their illnesses.

PRINCIPLES FOR SUCCESSFUL TRANSITION OF YACI

Transition services may be most successful in a nursing-led and managed transition care model, such as the one described by Betz and Redcay's[38] CHF program. The CHF model was originally designed to address the transition needs of adolescent and early YA aged 13 to 22 years, but because of the multiple unmet transition needs of adults, the services now support adults up to the age of 40 years. The CHF program makes use of existing community resources, which avoids duplication of services and assures that specific services are available. Community physicians, such as internists, may be more appropriate to address the recognition and prevention of chronic illness in YACCS as well as those YAs served by the CHF program. Community physicians or family physicians and internists can not only address the potential and realized late complications of childhood cancer treatment but also manage the health conditions of aging adults, such as hypertension, diabetes, and coronary heart disease. Although there is no evidence to suggest that this model is the most effective one, it may be the most cost-effective.

Betz and Redcay[23,37] first described their model for healthy transitions for YAs with chronic disease. The CHF program used evidence-based principles to guide the transition for the YA with special needs. Models of cancer transition may be tailored to meet the needs of YACCS, specifically survivors with an increased risk for delayed effects of cancer treatment later in life, similar to the approach used by Jacobs.[3,39] In their model, Betz and Redcay[23,37] described how the nurse played an integral role as the service coordinator, bridging the gaps between the pediatric and adult care models. An interdisciplinary, risk-focused approach to health care for the YACI, with nurses playing an important role in the transition of the YA, may be the most successful.

The responsibility for establishing appropriate transition services for AYA cancer survivors lies in the hands of the pediatric oncology center. Pediatric nurses and APNs are in the best position to influence and ascertain that the most appropriate and successful transition services are provided for survivors. As adolescent cancer survivors with chronic disease make their way through high school and college, services for students with disabilities are available.[24] The ownership of linking the survivors with disabilities to services lies with the pediatric nursing staffs who have worked with the YACCS who are entering college. Adult practitioners may not be aware of the multiple services available for children with disabilities. Therefore, the concept of a nurse-driven interdisciplinary model to provide formal transition of YACCS with chronic illness to adult services is warranted.

The CHF model uses a nurse-led approach to provide consultant services to transition adolescents to adult practices. The program takes into consideration the individual needs of the youth. Use of an interdisciplinary team has been successful in assuring that resources are available and provided to the AYA with special needs.[23,37] Templates can be developed to adapt this model of transition for YACCS with chronic illness to the most appropriate adult services. Because of the unique needs of YACI and YACCS with CNS tumors specifically,[34] a formal plan should be part of any successful transition model.

Researchers[42–44] proposed several elements for the successful transition of adolescents to adult services, including (1) recognizing that transition is another phase in health care treatment, (2) assessing and obtaining readiness in the YA, (3) providing coordination of services between pediatric and adult providers, and (4) making available training programs for professionals involved in the transition. In addition, professionals need to take into consideration the normal developmental tasks of adolescence so that the adolescents are able to acquire the necessary skills for a successful transition.[44] Health care should be financially accessible for AYAs and is imperative to ensure the availability of future health care services.[21]

Preparing the YA for transition requires several steps, one of which is preparing the YA to be independent and to be able to function in an adult care center.[44] Assessing readiness is the first step in preparing the adolescent before the actual transition to adult services as a YA. Another step is providing educational programs to educate adolescents about their disease and how to manage side effects, order medications, and make appointments. Other important skills include how to talk to adult practitioners and when and who to call in the event of a health crisis.[44] During the next phase of transition, meeting the adult provider in a safe environment may be useful to ensure communication between the pediatric and adult health care providers and the YA. Identifying several adult services willing and educated in the health care needs of YAs with childhood-onset chronic health needs is imperative to a successful long-term transition of health care. The administrative policy and support between the institutions or freestanding centers will go far to sustain a formal and successful transition of care.[43,44]

Nurses and pediatric practitioners are best able to provide adequate preparation of the AYA for more successful transition to independency. Nurturing the YA as well as the adult care provider is an important concept to ensure sustainability of the collaboration between the providers and to ensure appropriate health services for the YA. Listening to the AYAs' views on transition ensures a smooth and successful transition; this includes active participation in their own health care decisions; the provision of accessible information about services; the establishment of a shared philosophy between pediatric and adult services; honesty; advocacy for their needs; and consideration of the attitudes, behaviors, and uniqueness of the YA population.

SUMMARY

Transition for YACI and adolescents with special needs to adult services has been fraught with many obstacles. Historically, many children did not survive congenital illnesses or cancers and did not have the need for adult services with expertise in childhood chronic illness. Children now diagnosed with cancer are surviving long term and are at risk for developing late-onset chronic diseases. Transition services are being developed across the country. YACCS are not all adequately transitioned to adult services for many reasons. Pediatric nurses and advanced practitioners are the likely leaders in the movement of these YACCS from pediatric to adult centers.

REFERENCES

1. Hewitt M, Weiner SL, Somone JV, editors. Childhood cancer survivorship improving care and quality of life. Washington, DC: National Academies Press; 2003.
2. Oeffinger KC, Mertens AC, Sklar CA, et al. Chronic health conditions in adult survivors of childhood cancer. N Engl J Med 2006;355:1572–82.
3. Henderson TO, Friedman DL, Meadows AT. Childhood cancer survivors: transition to adult-focused risk-based care. Pediatrics 2010;126:129–36.
4. Schumacher KL, Meleis A. Transitions: a central concept in nursing. Image J Nurs Sch 1994;26:119–27.
5. MacLean WE, Foley GV, Ruccione K, et al. Transitions in the care of adolescent and young adult survivors of childhood cancer. Cancer 1996;78:1340–4.
6. Bridges W. Being in transition. In: Transitions: making sense of life's changes. 2nd edition. New York: De Capo Press; 2004. p. 1–24.
7. Kralik D, Visentin K, van Loon A. Transition: a literature review. J Adv Nurs 2006; 55:320–9.
8. Doulton DM. From cradle to commencement: transitioning pediatric sickle cell disease patients to adult providers. J Pediatr Oncol Nurs 2010;27:119–23.

9. Schidlow DV, Fiel SB. Life beyond pediatrics. Transition of chronically ill adolescents from pediatric to adult health care systems. Med Clin North Am 1990;74: 1113–20.

10. Kirk S. Transitions in the lives of young people with complex healthcare needs. Child Care Health Dev 2008;2008(34):567–75.

11. Sawyer SM, Drew S, Yeo MS, et al. Adolescents with a chronic condition: challenges living, challenges treating. Lancet 2007;369:1481–9.

12. Stam H, Hartman EE, Deurloo JA, et al. Young adult patients with a history of pediatric disease: impact on course of life and transition into adulthood. J Adolesc Health 2006;39:4–13.

13. Tuchman LK, Schwartz LA, Sawicki GS, et al. Cystic fibrosis and transition to adult medical care. Pediatrics 2010;125:566–73.

14. Tuchman LK, Slap GB, Britto MT. Transition to adult care: experiences and expectations of adolescents with chronic illness. Child Care Health Dev 2008;34:557–63.

15. Viner R. Bridging the gaps: transition for young people with cancer. Eur J Cancer 2003;39:2684–7.

16. Betz CL. Transition of adolescents with special health care needs: review and analysis of the literature. Issues Compr Pediatr Nurs 2004;27:179–241.

17. Sawyer SM. In search of quality care for adolescents and young adults with chronic conditions. J Paediatr Child Health 2008;44:475–7.

18. Reiss JG, Gibson RW, Walker LR. Health care transitions: youth, family and provider perspectives. Pediatrics 2005;115:112–20.

19. American Academy of Pediatrics, American Academy of Family Physicians, American College of Physicians-American Society of Internal Medicine. A consensus statement on health care transitions for young adults with special health care needs. Pediatrics 2002;110:1304–6.

20. Rosen DS, Blum RW, Britto M, et al. Transition to adult health care for adolescents and young adults with chronic conditions: position paper of the society for adolescent medicine. J Adolesc Health 2003;33(4):309–11.

21. English A, Park MJ, Shafer MA, et al. Health care reform and adolescents-An agenda for the lifespan: a position paper of the society for adolescent medicine. J Adolesc Health 2009;45(3):310–5.

22. Baines JM. Promoting better care: transition from child to adult services. Nurs Stand 2009;23:35–40.

23. Betz CL, Redcay G. Dimensions of the transition service coordinator role. J Spec Pediatr Nurs 2004;10:49–59.

24. Betz CL. Adolescents with chronic conditions: linkages to adult service systems. Pediatr Nurs 1999;25:473–6, 496–7.

25. Betz CL. Facilitating the transition of adolescents with chronic conditions from pediatric to adult health care and community settings. Issues Compr Pediatr Nurs 1998;21:97–115.

26. Lewis-Gary MD. Transitioning to adult health care facilities for young adults with a chronic condition. Pediatr Nurs 2001;27:521–4.

27. Jalkut MK, Allen PJ. Transition from pediatric to adult health care for adolescents with congenital heart disease: a review of the literature and clinical implications. Pediatr Nurs 2009;35:381–7.

28. Okumura MJ, Kerr EA, Cabana MD, et al. Physician views on barriers to primary care for young adults with childhood-onset chronic disease. Pediatrics 2009;125: e748–54.

29. Viner R. Barriers and good practice in transition from paediatric to adult care. J R Soc Med 2001;94(Suppl 40):2–5.

30. Diller L, Chow EJ, Gurney JG, et al. Chronic disease in the childhood cancer survivor study cohort: a review of published findings. J Clin Oncol 2009;27:2339–55.
31. Friedman DL, Whitton J, Leisenring W. Subsequent neoplasms in 5-year survivors of childhood cancer: the childhood cancer survivor study. J Natl Cancer Inst 2010;21:1083–95.
32. Bowers DC, Liu Y, Leisenring W. Late-occurring stroke among long-term survivors of childhood leukemia and brain tumors: a report from the childhood cancer survivor study. J Clin Oncol 2006;24:5277–82.
33. Ness KK, Morris EB, Nolan VG, et al. Physical performance limitations among adult survivors of childhood brain tumors. Cancer 2010;116:3034–44.
34. Eshelman-Kent D, Gilger E, Gallagher M. Transitioning survivors of central nervous system tumors: challenges for patients, families, and health care providers. J Pediatr Oncol Nurs 2009;26:280–94.
35. Suris JC, Michaud PA, Viner R. The adolescent with a chronic condition. Part I: developmental issues. Arch Dis Child 2004;89:938–42.
36. Schwartz SA, Drotar D. Health-related hindrance of personal goal pursuit and well-being of young adults with cystic fibrosis, pediatric cancer survivors, and peer without a history of chronic illness. J Pediatr Psychol 2009;34:954–65.
37. Betz CL, Redcay G. Lessons learned from providing transition services to adolescents with special health care needs. Issues Compr Pediatr Nurs 2002;25:129–49.
38. Betz CL, Redcay G. Creating healthy futures: an innovative nurse-managed transition clinic for adolescents and young adults with special health care needs. Pediatr Nurs 2003;29:25–30.
39. Jacobs LA, Hobbie WL. The living well after cancer program: an advanced practice model of care. Oncol Nurs Forum 2002;29:637–8.
40. Scal P, Evans T, Blozis S, et al. Trends in transition from pediatric to adult health care services for young adults with chronic conditions. J Adolesc Health 1999;24:259–64.
41. Mertens AC, Cotter KL, Foster BF, et al. Improving health care for adult survivors of childhood cancer: recommendations from a delphi panel of health policy experts. Health Policy 2004;69:169–78.
42. Kennedy A, Sloman F, Douglass JA, et al. Young people with chronic illness: the approach to transition. Intern Med J 2007;37:555–60.
43. Viner RM. Transition of care from paediatric to adult services: once part of improved health services for adolescents. Arch Dis Child 2008;93:160–3.
44. Viner R. Effective transition from paediatric to adult services. Hosp Med 2000;61:341–3.

Pediatric Sepsis and Multiorgan Dysfunction Syndrome: Progress and Continued Challenges

Kay Lawrence, RN, MSN, CCRN, CPN

KEYWORDS

- Pediatric • Sepsis • Multiorgan dysfunction • Shock
- Critical care

Pediatric sepsis and the multiorgan dysfunction, which may accompany it, remain a significant cause of morbidity and mortality in pediatric intensive care units (PICUs). Mortality rates from severe sepsis and septic shock have decreased because clinicians have become better at early recognition and because we have learned more about effective treatment of these conditions.[1–4] Multiorgan dysfunction syndrome (MODS) continues to be a significant cause of both morbidity and mortality of children in the PICUs.[1–4] In addition, many children may suffer long-term deleterious effects from the disease process and/or from the treatment associated with that disease process.[2] This article reviews the current knowledge about sepsis and MODS in pediatric patients and discusses the best treatment modalities while highlighting the critical aspects of nursing care for this vulnerable population.

Although MODS may result from numerous insults, such as trauma or burns, the concepts of multiorgan dysfunction associated with septic shock are a useful framework for understanding multiorgan dysfunction in general. The issues of sepsis, septic shock, and MODS are discussed further in terms of what is currently known about the ensuant pathophysiology, host response, and management strategies.

SHOCK

To communicate fluently about any topic we must first have the same understanding of the terminologies used. Shock, put most simply, is the inability of the body to supply

The author has nothing to disclose.
Pediatric Intensive Care Unit, Medical College of Georgia School of Nursing, Medical College of Georgia Children's Medical Center, 1446 Harper Street, BT3933, Augusta, GA 30912, USA
E-mail address: klawrence@georgiahealth.edu

adequate nutrients and oxygen to the cells.[4] There are 2 broad categories of shock: low flow and distributive shocks. These categories are further subdivided into hypovolemic and cardiogenic shocks, which are categorized as low flow shock, and septic, anaphylactic, and neurogenic shocks, which are categorized as distributive shock. A good working analogy for low flow shock is a train. There must be enough volume in the cars to supply the needs of the cells, but there must also be enough power in the engine to pull the cars around. In hypovolemic shock, there is simply not enough volume to supply the cells. In cardiogenic shock, the problem is with the engine. The cardiac muscle is damaged to the degree that it cannot push the volume where it needs to go.

Alternatively with distributive shock, the problem is less about volume and more about where that volume is going and if it is effective in delivering the needed materials to the cells. In anaphylactic and neurogenic shocks, there is significant vasodilation, which effectively increases the capacity of the vascular space. Without significantly increased volume, there is a relative intravascular hypovolemia.

A hallmark feature of septic shock is capillary leakage along with vasodilation, thus decreasing the relative intravascular volume. It is critical to understand that in terms of end-organ perfusion, it is the intravascular volume that counts. Regardless of how much volume there is in the interstitium, that volume is not helpful to the perfusion of end organs. So, with respect to septic shock, the problem is less about absolute volume but more about where that volume is. Other definitions pertinent to this discussion are presented in **Table 1**.

PATHOPHYSIOLOGY OF SEPSIS AND SEPTIC SHOCK

As previously discussed, shock is a final common pathway of many physiologic processes. With septic shock, there is an initial infection that triggers the immune response of the host. Common causative organisms vary by age and are summarized in **Box 1**. Infants and children are more susceptible to infection and sepsis because of differences in their anatomy, in their immune systems, and in their abilities to compensate.[2]

Table 1 Common terms associated with shock and MODS	
	Definitions
Bacteremia	The presence of bacteria in the blood
Sepsis	The presence of bacteremia with evidence of systemic inflammatory response and infection
Systemic Inflammatory Response	2 or more of the following: Hyperthermia or hypothermia (>38°C or <36°C), Tachycardia Tachypnea, Increased or decreased white blood cell count (>12,000 per mL or <4000 per mL) Bandemia (>10% bands)
Severe Sepsis	The presence of sepsis with organ dysfunction, poor perfusion, or hypotension
Septic Shock	Sepsis with continued hypotension and perfusion abnormalities even after adequate fluid resuscitation
MODS	The failure of 2 or more organ systems

Box 1
Causative organisms of sepsis by age

Neonates

    Escherichia coli

    Klebsiella

    Enterobacter

    Group B streptococci

Infants and children

    Streptococcus pneumoniae

    Neisseria meningitides

    Haemophilus influenza type b

    Staphylococcus aureus

    Group A streptococci

Data from Sparrow A, Willis F. Management of septic shock in childhood. Emerg Med Australas 2004;16:126; with permission.

Once the initial infection occurs, response by the host to the infecting organism follows. The triggers to this response are the endotoxins or exotoxins that the infecting organism releases. An endotoxin is a lipopolysaccharide released from the cell wall of gram-negative bacteria during cell lysis. Endotoxins can cause fever and leukopenia, as well as possible diarrhea and hemorrhagic shock because of their effect on the host immune system. Certain cells, such as macrophages and endothelial cells, recognize endotoxins and trigger the release of inflammatory mediators in an effort to combat the bacteria.[4]

An exotoxin is a protein synthesized by microorganisms including bacteria, fungi, algae, and protozoa. Exotoxins are found outside the bacterial wall. Released during growth of bacteria, exotoxins have very specific effects such as damage to cell membranes, inhibition of protein synthesis, and production of antibodies called antitoxins.[3,4] Contact with endotoxins and exotoxins causes the body to release several mediators, which may be divided into the broad categories of proinflammatory and anti-inflammatory mediators. Proinflammatory mediators include cytokines such as tumor necrosis factor, interleukins (ILs), thromboxane A_2, prostacyclin, platelet activating factor, and nitric oxide. Antiinflammatory mediators include lipopolysaccharide-binding protein, IL-1 receptor antagonist–soluble CD14, type 2 IL-1 receptor antagonist, and leukotriene B_4 receptor antagonist (**Fig. 1**).[3–6]

Although the human immune system is normally a well-oiled machine that works in a balance that is finely tuned, when the conditions of septic shock are present, the system is overloaded and out of balance, thus producing the many clinical manifestations that are seen in these patients.[3–6] These manifestations may include tachycardia, tachypnea, fever, poor perfusion, altered mental status, and other indications of organ dysfunction. Neonates in particular may exhibit different manifestations, such as hypothermia, instead of fever because of the immaturity of their immune systems. As organ failure progresses, manifestations may change along with clinical conditions in all patients.

The initial response of the immune system is weighted heavily in the favor of proinflammatory mediators, which produce the endothelial dysfunction that subsequently

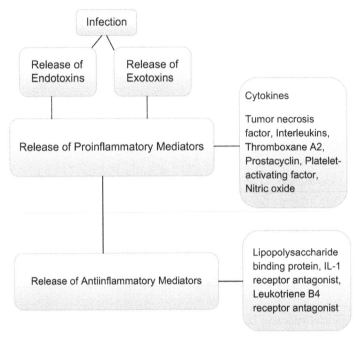

Fig. 1. Host response to initial infection.

leads to the hallmark feature of capillary leak. As the capillaries become more permeable to fluid, the intravascular volume leaks into the interstitial space while simultaneously vasodilation is producing reduced vascular resistance, causing a relative intravascular hypovolemia. Cardiac output may increase enough to compensate, so that the skin remains warm to touch and pink or even hyperemic. If the cardiac output cannot increase enough to compensate, the child may exhibit the more typical signs and symptoms of hypovolemia, including cool pale skin. The clinical presentation of these children frequently involves a history of a localized infection, eg, otitis media, upper respiratory tract infection, or urinary tract infection, which is then followed by a rapid decline to a cool mottled appearance, tachycardia, fever, and decreased level of consciousness. With some very aggressive organisms, such as the gram-negative bacteria, the hemodynamic decline is so rapid that caregivers do not notice the initial infection.

Without a doubt, the biggest concern in the clinical presentation of these children is cardiorespiratory failure. Cardiac output is a function of heart rate and stroke volume. Infants and children are less able to increase their stroke volume compared with adults making them depend on an increased heart rate to increase cardiac output to meet increased system demands. These increased demands are caused by the relative intravascular hypovolemia and also frequently by fever. The inability of the heart to meet these demands for increased output leads to other presenting signs and symptoms including poor perfusion. As the cells become unable to get enough oxygen to meet the body's demands, they switch over to anaerobic metabolism leading to lactic acid buildup and acidosis. The lack of oxygen and the acidotic environment also contribute to the failure of the sodium/potassium pump in the cell walls, leading to electrolyte imbalances that may further compromise the ability of the myocardium to respond.[3,4]

MODS

Inadequate cardiac output, along with the showers of proinflammatory and antiinflammatory mediators, can further progress to multiorgan dysfunction. Multiorgan dysfunction may be thought of as the failure of 2 or more organ systems in the presence of acute illness when homeostasis cannot be maintained without intervention.[1,7] Cardiac output decreases because of vasodilation and capillary leakage, which in turn affects the intravascular volume and the inability of the myocardial muscle to meet demand. Lactic acidosis develops when cells must switch to anaerobic metabolism. The acidotic environment results in electrolyte imbalances, which in turn may further decrease the cardiac output. Simultaneously, other organ systems are affected by the lack of oxygen and glucose, by the buildup of lactic acid, and by capillary leakage.

Another mechanism of inflammation may be the process of apoptosis.[1] When a cell lives its normal life span and then dies, it causes no disturbance to other cells, a process known as apoptosis. When necrotic (or oxygen-deprived) cells die, they can cause an inflammatory response. In MODS, cells basically undergo apoptosis and necrotic death at an accelerated rate. The process of apoptosis and the varying ways that organs modulate this process has been postulated as a way to explain the order of organ system failure in adults.[1] Although the body is a complex interaction of all organ systems, the systems will be considered on an individual basis.

Neurologic System

The brain is often one of the first organ systems affected by sepsis. Septic encephalopathy may be difficult to diagnose in the clinical setting because so many other things are going on simultaneously and many of the necessary interventions could cloud the neurologic picture. Children often present with an altered level of consciousness, which may be related to fatigue, fever, or hypovolemia.[3,4] In addition, there may be some disturbance in the blood-brain barrier, which is ordinarily a protective mechanism that regulates the cerebral environment very tightly. The mechanism for the disruption of this barrier may be related to changes in the microcirculation in response to inflammatory mediators, leading to many small areas of ischemia.[8] The brain requires high levels of oxygen and glucose in normal circumstances in any shock state, but more particularly with septic shock, in which that requirement is increased at a time when the heart is already having trouble providing adequate output. So, the decreased level of consciousness seen in children with septic shock and concomitant neurologic dysfunction may be a function of lack of oxygen and glucose and may also be related to disruption of the blood-brain barrier in response to inflammatory mediators.[8]

Respiratory System

The respiratory system is most often the system in a child that gets attention in a hurry in the emergency department or the PICU. The child with septic shock often presents with respiratory distress or failure, requiring immediate and expert management. Respiratory distress is recognized in the child who has increased work of breathing but is able to maintain acid-base balance. In respiratory failure, the child is no longer able to compensate and may have very shallow and infrequent respirations, which are ineffective in removing enough carbon dioxide (CO_2) to maintain the pH within normal limits. In children with septic shock, there are several processes taking place (most notably capillary leak) that may cause a progression to acute lung injury (ALI) or acute respiratory distress syndrome (ARDS). ALI/ARDS may be caused by several different problems from trauma to aspiration, but septic shock seems to be a frequently seen trigger.[3,9] A commonly accepted definition of ALI/ARDS is that of the American European Consensus Conference and includes acute onset, severe hypoxemia refractory to oxygen therapy, diffuse pulmonary infiltrates, and no evidence of left-sided heart failure.[9] The difference between ALI and ARDS is the degree of hypoxemia, with ALI being defined as a Pao_2/fraction of inspired oxygen (Fio_2) ratio less than 40 kPa and ARDS being defined as a Pao_2/Fio_2 ratio less than 26.7 kPa.[10]

The mechanism of lung injury is related to capillary leak, endothelial damage, and the inflammatory response. Capillary leakage within the pulmonary vasculature causes fluid to leak from the capillaries to the interstitial spaces, creating a gap between the alveoli and the capillaries, making diffusion of oxygen and carbon dioxide more difficult. Fluid may migrate from this interstitial space into the alveolar space, further compromising diffusion and causing alveolar consolidation. There is also a migration of various cells into the alveolar space, further impairing diffusion. The type II alveolar cells no longer make surfactant, causing the alveoli to close down at the end of expiration and become more difficult to reopen. It was this mechanism that caused ARDS to be first called so because of the perceived similarities to neonatal respiratory distress syndrome in which the lack of surfactant production is a major feature. And, as if all this were not enough, platelet aggregation in the pulmonary capillaries causes obstruction of these capillaries, contributing further to capillary leak and further disturbing pulmonary perfusion.[1]

The Cardiovascular System

The cardiovascular system is affected by all of the same mediators as the other systems in the body. Although hypoperfusion of the myocardium and low intravascular volume explain myocardial dysfunction to a degree, there is more to the story. It seems that impairment of the contractile apparatus of the cardiac muscle may play a large role. With sepsis, both the ability to contract (inotropy) and the ability to relax (chronotropy) may be affected by regulating proteins, which are in turn affected by various mediators. In adults, MODS-related death is often caused by vasomotor paralysis, whereas in children, low cardiac output caused by myocardial dysfunction is often the cause of MODS-related death.[9] This dysfunction seems to be unrelated to changes in vascular resistance and requires a different approach to diagnosis and treatment.[9] Pediatric patients should continue to be evaluated and their treatment guided by vigilant assessment including the assessment of perfusion as well as vital signs. In general, the pediatric patient evidences changes in peripheral circulation by developing mottled, cool extremities. Mental status and peripheral perfusion should remain the mainstays of assessment, and initial therapies should be directed at restoring peripheral perfusion. It is important that the critical care nurse understand that when skin temperature and capillary refill are assessed, the assumption lies that if the skin is well perfused, other end organs are well perfused. The body preserves flow to the heart, brain, lungs, kidneys, and other organs in preference to the skin.[6]

Technologies are available to more accurately assess cardiac index, stroke volume index, systemic vascular resistance index, global end-diastolic index, and extravascular lung water index. A complete discussion of these monitoring devices is beyond the scope of this article, but readers should be aware that pulse contour analysis and ultrasonic technologies are available to take the place of the pulmonary artery catheter in small patients. The newer technologies are noninvasive or much less invasive when compared with pulmonary artery catheters, and continued improvements are expected to be seen in the future.[11–14]

An additional cardiovascular aspect of septic shock includes endogenous catacholamines. In normal states, endogenous vasopressin acts synergistically with the rennin-angiotensin-aldosterone system to regulate blood pressure. With septic shock, the levels of endogenous vasopressin may be depleted; therefore, administering physiologic doses of vasopressin may help to maintain the child's blood pressure.[15]

Renal System

The renal system performs important functions in terms of fluid and electrolyte balance, acid-base balance, and blood pressure regulation. To perform these functions, the kidneys must receive adequate perfusion and the endocrine system must function appropriately. In general, renal failure is divided into 3 basic types: prerenal, intrarenal, and postrenal. Prerenal failure is often caused by poor perfusion to the kidneys, so that the kidneys lack not only oxygen and glucose but also fluid to filter. Intrarenal failure is often caused by poor perfusion to the renal tubules, resulting in acute tubular necrosis. Postrenal failure is caused by some form of obstruction leading to hydronephrosis.[16]

With septic shock, in which the cardiac output is poor, intravascular volume is inadequate and cellular debris or platelet aggregation may cause obstruction in the small capillaries. In the past, it was thought that the kidneys were underperfused, leading to acute tubular necrosis; however, histologic evidence in postmortem studies now suggests that the kidneys remain well perfused in septic shock.[16] There is local production of nitric oxide, which leads to vasodilation, suggesting that the renal perfusion may actually increase. More pertinent causes for acute renal failure in septic shock and MODS may include inflammation with the release of proinflammatory and antiinflammatory mediators. The role of apoptosis and necrotic cell death is less clear at this time.[16]

Gastrointestinal Tract

It has long been thought that sepsis and MODS disrupt the mucosal barrier of the gut, allowing migration of bacteria, endotoxins, and exotoxins into the portal vein, thereby worsening the overall illness.[4] Although it is less sure that this is the mechanism, there remains some certainty that the gut is hypoperfused and that this may lead to stress ulcers and even ileus. The liver plays an important role in the clearance of various toxins from the body. It is also active in the production of various proinflammatory mediators. The liver seems to be somewhat less directly affected by sepsis. Some possible reasons for this may be the tremendous reserve that the liver has or its high level of antioxidants, which perform a protective function.[1,16]

Endocrine System

The endocrine system is perhaps the most complex and least understood organ system within the body. Much has been written in the adult literature about tight glycemic control.[17,18] In pediatrics, there is less research, and so the risks and benefits of tight glucose control are less well understood. Some research suggests that prevention of hyperglycemia (blood glucose level >126 mg/dL) may be beneficial in patients with 3 or more organ systems in clinical failure.[16] Hypoglycemia, at the other end of the spectrum, was also associated with longer PICU and hospital lengths of stay.[17] In addition, the relationship of blood glucose level, insulin administration, and recovery involves the somatotropic axis,[19] which consists of the pituitary gland, cerebral cortex, hypothalamus, kidney, liver, and limbic system.

In a complex series of events, growth hormone and insulin-like growth factors I and II are released during catabolism of protein.[20] In individuals with normal physiology, these hormones stimulate the synthesis of protein and stop the muscle wasting that may occur in catabolic states. In sepsis and MODS, it seems that proinflammatory cytokines may alter somatotropic axis function. This alteration may result in an imbalance in multiple hormones and regulatory proteins. Animal studies suggest that growth hormone is less effective in resistant states, such as critical illness.[19–21] Tight glucose control is also implicated as a factor causing poor response to growth hormone.[7,16] The effects associated with the endocrine system in children with sepsis are extremely complex, and research in this area is still fairly new, so our understanding of the complex interactions is incomplete to say the least. Future directions will no doubt reveal much more about the endocrine aspects of sepsis, septic shock, and MODS.[19]

Disseminated Intravascular Coagulation

Disseminated intravascular coagulation (DIC) has long been recognized as a prognosticator of poor outcome in patients with sepsis, systemic inflammatory response syndrome (SIRS), and MODS. The trigger for DIC seems to be the same as that of other organ dysfunctions in MODS and SIRS, although the presence of intravascular fibrin or coagulation proteases may be involved in determining the patient's clinical course. Although it has traditionally been thought that gram-negative sepsis made one more susceptible to DIC, gram-positive organisms can certainly cause DIC as well.[21] Whereas the normal coagulation cascade usually proceeds in an orderly manner, in the child with sepsis, SIRS, and MODS, this changes. Fibrinolysis is impaired, so fibrin is not removed from the plasma and fibrinogenesis occurs to a greater degree. Generation of thrombin is increased and there is a simultaneous suppression of anticoagulation, thus upsetting the balance of coagulation/anticoagulation that is normally present in the body. Proinflammatory cytokines begin this cascade by increasing levels of thrombin, which converts fibrinogen to fibrin. Cytokines also cause levels of antithrombin III (ATIII) to be low, the function of protein C to be impaired, and low amounts of tissue factor pathway inhibitor to be present. All these mechanisms result in excessive fibrin, which in turn causes thrombi to form and wedge in small vessels. There is no single definitive laboratory test for DIC; so multiple tests are used along with clinical assessment. Laboratory tests include prothrombin time (PT), activated partial thromboplastin time (aPTT), platelet level, ATIII levels, and levels of other factor.

The criteria for a diagnosis of DIC include presence of a disease process known to cause DIC, platelet count of less than 100,000 or a falling platelet count, prolonged PT or aPTT, and low levels of ATIII. Severe liver dysfunction may result in the same laboratory values because DIC and fibrinogen levels may initially be normal, so it is important to consider the patient's overall clinical picture when diagnosing DIC. Classically, DIC is exhibited by a hypercoagulation phase followed by a stage of inadequate coagulation and bleeding. It is difficult to know when a patient is in a hypercoagulation state, making DIC sometimes noted when the child begins to show clinical signs of poor clotting. Often these clinical signs include bleeding from intravenous (IV) or central line sites and bleeding from very vascular tissues such as the gums or nose or within the gastrointestinal tract.[3,21]

TREATMENT OF SEPSIS, SEPTIC SHOCK, AND MODS

Treatment of sepsis, septic shock, and MODS can be divided into 2 phases, early and late. Any child with an infection may present with fever, tachycardia, and vasodilation. Children who present with an alteration in their mental status should provoke a high degree of suspicion of septic shock.[1,5,16] Treatment during the early phase consists of cardiorespiratory stabilization and initiation of broad-spectrum antibiotic therapy.

The first action is to assess and secure the airway, ensure gas exchange, and assess the child's cardiac status. The experienced practitioner is quickly tuned into the signs and symptoms of severe respiratory distress or failure. If children seem to be unable to maintain an airway, they should be endotracheally intubated by a skilled practitioner. Positive pressure ventilation is then initiated via bag valve mask or mechanical ventilation.

The initiation of positive pressure ventilation has the effect of increasing intrathoracic pressure, which in turn increases pressure on the vena cava. This increase reduces venous return to the right atrium and preload, which in turn decreases the cardiac output. The patient whose perfusion status has been tenuous may have a decrease in blood pressure and/or a compromise in perfusion, requiring additional crystalloids.[5,6] Trends in ventilation have migrated toward smaller tidal volumes (Vts) (7–8 mL/kg) to prevent ventilator-associated lung injury (VALI).[5,6] Once the airway is secured and ventilation initiated, arterial or capillary blood gases are obtained to assist with management of ventilator settings. The management goal is to normalize the pH and Pco_2 as much as possible without causing barotraumas to the lungs.[5,6]

Once the airway is secured and ventilation initiated, perfusion is assessed. If perfusion is compromised, the child should receive a bolus of 20 mL/kg of crystalloid fluid. Fluid boluses are repeated at 20 mL/kg until perfusion is restored (capillary refill of <2 seconds) or until at least 60 mL/kg has been given.[5] It should be emphasized that adequate fluid volume is critical to support perfusion; so if it is not possible to quickly obtain IV access, intraosseous access should be obtained and initial fluid resuscitation started through that device. This alternative not only saves time but also saves veins until the child is better hydrated and until peripheral venous access is more likely to be successful.

The fluid of choice for initial resuscitation continues to be normal saline, although there are little research data regarding appropriate fluids for fluid resuscitation.[22] It is thought that approximately 25% of crystalloid solutions remain in the vascular space, whereas the other 75% leaks out into the interstitial space so that the intravascular volume is increased only on a short-term basis.[22] So frequently, clinicians find themselves giving up to 100 mL/kg of normal saline and observing the patient becoming more edematous because they struggle to maintain the intravascular volume. It is helpful to remember at this point in treatment that the volume that counts is the intravascular volume. Later on in treatment, as the patient improves, the fluid that is going into the interstitial space will return to the vascular space and can be eliminated with the aid of diuretics or renal replacement therapy, if necessary.

Although it seems logical that hypertonic saline or a colloid solution, such as hetastarch or albumin, might reduce the migration of fluids out of the vascular space, few studies have been performed to research the efficacy of these fluids. If, after 3 boluses of crystalloid solution, the child's blood pressure does not increase and perfusion remains compromised, the use of inotropic agents must be considered. Hypoglycemia and hypocalcemia must be corrected. Once these 2 parameters are corrected and preload has increased, more attention must be directed toward the use of inotropic agents to support circulation.

Fluid refractory shock refers to shock that does not respond to fluid resuscitation.[5] If perfusion is not corrected with 60 mL or more per kilogram; dopamine is started as a first-line inotropic agent in the presence of low systemic vascular resistance. Dobutamine is an additional first-line option in the presence of increased systemic vascular resistance. Other agents that may be used are epinephrine, norepinephrine, and vasopressin. In the case of adequate blood pressure and increased systemic or pulmonary vascular resistance, milrinone may be added to improve peripheral perfusion. The goal of therapy is an adequate blood pressure with adequate peripheral perfusion and a cardiac index of 3.3 to 6 L per minute per meter squared of the body surface area.[1,5,6]

All members of the critical care team should be aware that septic shock is an extremely dynamic process and that the patient's clinical status can and will change from minute to minute. The medication that does wonders for perfusion 1 minute may not be as effective 5 minutes later. Close observation and skilled assessment are critical for the appropriate use of these powerful pharmaceutical agents. Another consideration for children receiving pharmacotherapy is that the patient's response may be altered because of septic shock and MODS. The liver and kidneys are not functioning normally, which may cause elimination to be altered. Guidelines for choosing an appropriate dose for inotropic agents are just that, guidelines for a starting point. Each patient's dose must be titrated to his or her individual clinical response.

Antibiotics should be initiated as quickly as possible in cases of suspected sepsis. Once culture and sensitivity reports are received on any specimens sent, antibiotic therapy can be more finely adjusted. If all cultures give negative results, broad-spectrum antibiotics should be discontinued.[2,5,19] The death of bacterial cells results in the release of endotoxins, which stimulate the immune system; this in turn results in the release of inflammatory mediators, which are responsible for the body's response to the overwhelming infection. This is the same process that causes MODS to begin with. When antibiotics are administered, large numbers of bacterial cells die, releasing large amounts of endotoxins all at once. The critical care nurse should be aware that the patient's condition may actually worsen with the first dose of antibiotics and be prepared to rebolus with the fluid of choice or begin/increase inotropic support.

Once initial resuscitation is well underway, blood, sputum, and urine cultures are obtained; antibiotics are started; and long-term management is considered. The management of MODS will subsequently be discussed by system; however, one should remain aware of the close interaction of all body systems in patients affected by this condition. The treatment of MODS requires constant vigilance and skilled communication to balance the many issues under consideration. The patient with MODS is likely to be the most complex patient in the PICU and requires the best efforts of all team members.

Neurologic System

With respect to the neurologic system, the goal is to optimize oxygen delivery and minimize cerebral oxygen demands by decreasing cerebral metabolism. To do this, the child should have adequate oxygenation, optimal sedation, neuromuscular blockade, if necessary, maintenance of euthermia, and minimal stimulation. Oxygenation will be further addressed in the following section on respiratory system. The child who is critically ill and undergoing frightening and painful procedures should have adequate analgesia and anxiolysis. If it is necessary to use neuromuscular blockade, analgesia and anxiolysis become more imperative. The child's level of sedation must be assessed frequently, and there are several tools available to standardize assessment of sedation and pain relief.[23] In addition, as the patient's condition warrants, there should be a drug holiday instituted daily. A drug holiday consists of discontinuing neuromuscular blockade until slight movement is noted, then it is restarted. Keeping the room quiet, providing soft music, and providing a favorite soft blanket may help with control of anxiety and cerebral metabolism. Control of fever with acetaminophen, ibuprofen, and/or cooling devices can help control cerebral metabolism as well.

Respiratory System

Once initial resuscitation is accomplished and the child is intubated and placed on mechanical ventilation with initial settings, the focus shifts to optimizing gas exchange while minimizing VALI. In most cases, the initial F_{IO_2} is set at 1.00 and weaned from there as quickly as possible. Oxygen is a powerful drug with deleterious side effects and like any other drug, should be administered in a minimally effective dose. In the diagnosis of ARDS, the key feature is refractory hypoxemia; because of this, an attempt is made to keep the arterial oxygen saturation levels at greater than 92% in children with no preexisting conditions.[10] There are times, however, that 90% or even 88% may be accepted to avoid complications.

The next issue to consider is the child's $Paco_2$ levels. The parameters that may be manipulated to increase CO_2 removal are primarily rate and Vt and, to a lesser degree, positive end-expiratory pressure (PEEP). The goal for patients with ARDS is the maintenance of a normal $Paco_2$ (range of 35–45); however, this maintenance is often not possible, and frequently, permissive hypercapnia is practiced in which a $Paco_2$ of more than 50 mmHg is accepted to avoid lung injury due to barotrauma (trauma related to pressure).[10]

Another important consideration in the respiratory management of ALI and ARDS is alveolar recruitment. The presence of extra fluid and cells in the alveoli can cause consolidation and inability to ventilate those alveoli. Loss of surfactant can cause alveolar collapse and difficulty in opening alveoli on inspiration. If alveoli are recruited too forcefully, they may be injured in the process called atelectrauma (trauma related to the surfaces of the alveoli rubbing together while being popped open during inspiration). PEEP is still a mainstay in the treatment of ALI/ARDS, with the goal being to optimize PEEP to keep alveoli open while avoiding barotraumas or atelectrauma. An alternate method of ventilation is high-frequency oscillatory ventilation (HFOV). A complete discussion of ventilatory strategies is beyond the scope of this article but very briefly, HFOV essentially stents the airway open and gas exchange occurs around this stent. Oxygenation and ventilation are separated, making management of one somewhat independent of the other.[10]

Cardiovascular System

Skilled cardiovascular management is essential for children who have MODS. Vascular volume, cardiac output, and both systemic and pulmonary vascular resistances must be optimized. The use of various inotropic, chronotropic, and vasodilating agents is common in the intensive care units. We must always be aware, however, that nothing comes without a price. These drugs are very powerful and cause stress to the myocardium. Again, minimally effective dosages are essential. Having protocols in place for nurses to titrate drips at the bedside can assist in avoiding delays in the adjustment of these medications for optimal effect. As always, excellent and frequent communication among team members is critical.[3–6,11]

Renal Management

Renal failure is often a component of MODS. The child who initially presents with septic shock may have high serum urea nitrogen because of dehydration. If the serum urea nitrogen does not correct with adequate rehydration, the creatinine level increases to 2 times the patient's baseline, and/or other electrolyte abnormalities are present, the child is considered to have acute renal failure. Treatment is aimed at supporting the patient until the kidneys can recover. If the renal failure is mild, diuretics may be helpful. If renal failure is more severe, renal replacement therapies must be considered. The 2 modalities that are used for renal replacement therapy are hemodialysis and continuous venovenous hemodialysis (CVVH). The major advantage to both therapies is that vascular access can be obtained at the bedside. A major disadvantage to both therapies is that large bore catheters are necessary, which are challenging, if not impossible, to place in infants and small children.

Hemodialysis offers the ability to quickly and efficiently manage electrolyte abnormalities; however, it results in more drastic fluid shifts, often necessitating replacement of fluid that was removed too quickly. CVVH requires much more time and expertise for the critical care nurse to initiate and manage; however, it allows for electrolyte correction more slowly, removes fluid at a steady rate, and is usually better tolerated by small, very sick patients.[24] In either case, parents and caregivers require expert explanation with frequent reinforcement of information because it is understandably frightening to see their child's blood volume circulating outside the body.

Gastrointestinal System

Early enteral feedings have become standard in many conditions including sepsis, septic shock, and MODS. Although newer research casts some doubt on bacterial translocation by way of the portal vein,[1,16] it is thought anecdotally that the gut recovers better when fed at least at a trophic rate. Many centers feed patients transpylorically with the theory that chances of aspiration are lessened.[25]

Hepatic failure leads to DIC because the liver is the major organ that produces and regulates coagulation factors. DIC is still difficult to diagnose and treat. The pertinent laboratory tests were identified earlier in this discussion. Treatment of DIC is supportive and consists largely of transfusion of appropriate blood products as needed. These products include platelets, fresh frozen plasma, and cryoprecipitate.[21]

Endocrine System

The endocrine system is probably the most complex and least understood at present, although future research will no doubt elucidate the complexities of the endocrine system's response to sepsis, shock, and MODS. Blood glucose levels should be regulated to avoid hyperglycemia or hypoglycemia; however, the benefits of very tight glucose control in children are not clear. A stress dose of corticosteroids may be helpful for children who are at risk for adrenal insufficiency, including children with adrenal, hypothalamic, or pituitary disease, as well as those with a recent history of steroid usage. Any benefit to the use of multiple doses of steroids is not as clear. Although initially thought to be helpful, recent research is less conclusive.[26] Children who do not recover function of their somatotropic axis have been shown to have a higher mortality rate.[19] Future research will no doubt continue to elucidate the finer points of endocrine management in the setting of sepsis, septic shock, and MODS.

Nursing Care of the Child with Septic Shock and MODS

There is no factor more crucial to the survival of the pediatric patient with MODS than expert nursing care. Those children in whom sepsis is quickly recognized and treated have a lower risk of developing multiorgan failure.[27] Ongoing, vigilant, and expert assessment is crucial in identifying complications early, in administering therapies most effectively, and in monitoring the intended effects and adverse effects of these therapies. The roles of the critical care nurse may be thought of in terms of administering, monitoring, preventing, and teaching. The administration of various therapies requires technical expertise in several distinct technologies and vigilance in the application of these technologies. Various monitoring devices, multiple infusions, and medications must be balanced. The nurse is the last line of defense between the child and an error; therefore, hypervigilance is needed in checking and double checking everything that is done for that child.

All therapies must be monitored, and the information provided by technology should be correlated with the clinical picture. The nurse must interpret these data and communicate them effectively to other members of the critical care team. The nurse is also in a unique position to prevent potential complications. Children with septic shock and MODS are vulnerable to iatrogenic harm such as hospital-acquired infections, equipment malfunctions, and skin breakdown. Care bundles, such as those for ventilator-associated pneumonia, catheter-associated urinary tract infections, and blood stream infections are valuable resources that help the nurse to focus care on those interventions that are most useful in preventing complications.

Good basic nursing care, including turning the patient, and providing skin care help to protect these vulnerable children from skin breakdown. Perhaps the most important role of the nurse is teaching. Families are often devastated by a sudden illness that threatens the life of their child. The critical care nurse is in a unique position to educate and support families by explaining the child's condition, the therapies being instituted, what is hoped to be accomplished with those therapies, and how their child is responding. Caring is an important aspect of nursing, and should be communicated to family members as the nurse cares for their child.[28]

SUMMARY

Sepsis, septic shock, SIRS, and MODS remain clinical challenges in pediatric critical care. Understanding of the immune response has increased greatly over the past decade, which has certainly increased the understanding of the pathophysiology and treatment of these conditions. The future promises more exciting discoveries as we understand cellular physiology, immunity, and host responses even better. The treatment of sepsis, septic shock, SIRS, and most notably MODS remains complex, requiring the best of the art and science of all disciplines involved in the care of critically ill children as we strive to balance the treatment of multiple organ systems to the good of the whole child. To quote a great twentieth century philosopher who also loved children:

So be sure when you step, step with care and great tact, and remember that life's a great balancing act. Just never forget to be dexterous and deft. And never mix up your right foot with your left.[29]

—Dr Seuss

REFERENCES

1. Despond O, Proulx F, Carcillo J, et al. Pediatric sepsis and multiple organ dysfunction syndrome. Curr Opin Pediatr 2001;12:247–53.
2. Wynn J, Cornell T, Wong H, et al. The host response to sepsis and developmental impact. Pediatrics 2010;125(5):1031–41.
3. Hazinski MF. Shock, multiple organ dysfunction syndrome, and burns in children. In: McCance K, Huether S, editors. Pathophysiology: the biologic basis for disease in adults and children. 5th edition. St Louis (MO): Elsevier Mosby; 2006. p. 1655–80.
4. Sparrow A, Willis F. Management of septic shock in childhood. Emerg Med Australas 2004;16:125–34.
5. Brierley J, Carcillo J, Choong K, et al. Clinical practice parameters for hemodynamic support of pediatric and neonatal septic shock: 2007 update from the American college of critical care medicine. Crit Care Med 2009;37:666–88.

6. Carcillo J, Fields A. Clinical practice parameters for hemodynamic support of pediatric and neonatal patients in shock. Crit Care Med 2002;30:1365–77.
7. Proulx F, Joyal J, Mariscalco M. The pediatric multiple organ dysfunction syndrome. Pediatr Crit Care Med 2009;10:12–22.
8. Pytel P, Alexander J. Pathogenesis of septic encephalopathy. Curr opin neurol 2009;22:283–7.
9. Lorts A, Burroughs T, Shanley T. Elucidating the role of reversible protein phosphorylation in sepis-induced myocardial dysfunction. Shock 2009;32:49–54.
10. Randolph A. Management of acute lung injury and acute respiratory distress syndrome in children. Crit Care Med 2009;37:2448–54.
11. Cecchetti C, Lubrano R, Cristaldi S, et al. Relationship between global end-diastolic volume and cardiac output in critically ill infants and children. Crit Care Med 2008;36:928–32.
12. Wan L, Naka T, Uchino S, et al. A pilot study of pulse contour cardiac output monitoring in patients with septic shock. Crit Care Resusc 2005;7:160–5.
13. Berkowitz D, Danai P, Eaton S. Accurate characterization of extravascular lung water in acute respiratory distress syndrome. Crit Care Med 2008;36:1803–9.
14. Pauli C, Fakler U, Genz T. Cardiac output determination in children: equivalence of the transpulmonary thermodilution method to the direct Fick principle. Intensive Care Med 2002;28:947–52.
15. Ruggerio M. Effects of vasopressin in septic shock. AACN Adv Crit Care 2008;19:281–7.
16. Abraham E, Singer M. Mechanisms of sepsis-induced organ dysfunction. Crit Care Med 2007;35:2408–16.
17. Moghissi E. Reexamining the evidence for inpatient glucose control: new recommendations for glycemic targets. Am J Health Syst Pharm 2010;67(16 Suppl 8):S3–8.
18. Badawi O, Yeung S, Rosenfeld B. Evaluation of glycemic control metrics for intensive care unit populations. Am J Med Qual 2009;24(4):310–20.
19. Marquardt D, Knatz N, Wettarau L. Failure to recover somatotropic axis function is associated with mortality from pediatric sepsis-induced multiple organ dysfunction syndrome. Pediatr Crit Care Med 2010;11:18–25.
20. Mesotten D, Wouters P, Peeters R, et al. Regulation of the somatotropic axis by intensive insulin therapy during protracted critical illness. J Clin Endocrinol Metab 2004;89:3105–13.
21. Levi M, Ten-Cate H. Current concepts: disseminated intravascular coagulation. N Engl J Med 1999;341:587–92.
22. Akech A, Ledermann H, Maitland K. Choice of fluids for resuscitation in children with severe infection and shock: systematic review. BMJ 2010;341:c4416.
23. Curley M, Harris S, Fraser K, et al. State behavioral scale (SBS) a sedation assessment instrument for infants and young children supported on mechanical ventilation. Pediatr Crit Care Med 2006;7(2):107–14.
24. Van Biesen W, Vanholder R, Lameire N. Dialysis strategies in critically ill acute renal failure patients. Curr Opin Crit Care 2003;9(6):491–5.
25. Meert K, Daphtary K, Metheny N. Gastric vs small-bowel feeding in critically ill children receiving mechanical ventilation. Chest 2004;126(3):872–8.
26. Zimmerman J. A history of adjunctive glucocorticoid treatment for pediatric sepsis: moving beyond steroid pulp fiction toward evidence-based medicine. Pediatr Crit Care Med 2007;8:530–9.

27. Trzeciak S, McCoy J, Dellinger R. Early increases in microcirculatory perfusion during protocol-directed resuscitation are associated with reduced multi-organ failure at 24 h in patients with sepsis. Intensive Care Med 2008;34:2210–7.
28. Aldridge M. Decreasing parental stress in the pediatric intensive care unit: one unit's experience. Crit Care Nurse 2005;25:40–50.
29. Seuss D. Oh the places you'll go. New York: Random House; 1999.

Transcatheter Device Closure for Atrial Septal Defects: Safety, Efficacy, Complications, and Costs

Lindy Moake, RN, MSN, PCCNP*,
Samuel K. Ndinjiakat, RCIS, MSPAS, PA-C

KEYWORDS

- Congenital heart disease • Atrial septal defect
- Transcatheter closure • Atrial septal defect occlusion • Child

Congenital heart disease (CHD) is the most common birth defect known, occurring in 8 of 1000 live births.[1,2] Atrial septal defects (ASDs) are among the most common congenital cardiac defects seen by pediatric cardiologists and occur in 7% to 10% of all patients with congenital heart disease.[2,3] They often occur in conjunction with other cardiac defects and are known to occur twice as frequently in girls than in boys.[1,2] The presence of an ASD creates a communication between the left and right atrium, which allows blood to shunt from the higher pressure left atrium to the lower pressure right atrium. In time, this additional blood volume can result in enlargement of the right atrium and right ventricle and consequently results in increased pulmonary blood flow.[2,3] Most patients with ASDs have few symptoms.[2,3] Only 7% of patients with ASDs develop heart failure or require medications.[2] The most common complaints are fatigue and shortness of breath. Occasionally, children may have poor growth and multiple respiratory infections, but most are generally well. Patients with this defect are usually not diagnosed in infancy, but present as an asymptomatic child with a murmur. A cardiac examination, coupled with an electrocardiogram (ECG), chest radiograph, echocardiogram, and sometimes a cardiac catheterization, are key to confirming the diagnosis.

The authors have nothing to disclose.
Heart Center, Children's Medical Center of Dallas, 1935 Medical District Drive, Dallas, TX 75235, USA
* Corresponding author.
E-mail address: lindy.moake@childrens.com

Twenty percent of ASDs close spontaneously in the first year of life.[2] One percent of patients become symptomatic in the first year of life, with an associated 0.1% mortality.[2] If left unrepaired, ASDs have a lifetime mortality risk of 25% caused by many years of right ventricular volume overload that results in thickening of the pulmonary arteries leading to the development of a condition known as pulmonary hypertension. This volume overload is also associated with left ventricular distortion and dysfunction secondary to altered chamber geometry and decreased myofibril preload.[4] The recognition of these potential developments is the reason for elective closure of ASDs that have not spontaneously closed by school-age.[2]

ANATOMY AND PHYSIOLOGY OF ASDS

The atrial septum is composed of 2 septa, septum primum and septum secundum. The atrial septum divides the right and left atria and extends from the cavoatrial junction with the superior and inferior vena cava to the atrioventricular (AV) canal septum near the tricuspid valve.[4] There are 4 types of ASDs and their locations along the septum determine their types.

Sinus venosus ASDs occur at the junction of the superior vena cava and high atrial septum. These defects can be associated with anomalous drainage of the pulmonary veins.[5] Coronary sinus–type ASDs are located in the roof of the coronary sinus between its wall and the left atrium. Ostium primum ASDs are part of the spectrum of AV canal defects and are frequently associated with abnormalities of the AV valves.[3] These occur when the septum primum fails to complete its growth downward toward the atrioventricular valves.

Ostium secundum ASD is by far the most common anatomic type and the only true ASD.[4] Ostium secundum–type ASD represents approximately 80% of ASDs. It is centrally located in the region of the fossa ovalis along the atrial septum. This type of defect occurs when there is an insufficient amount of septal tissue. A recent study of this type of ASD in 104 children indicated that two-thirds of these defects continued to grow with time.[2] There is a similar defect located in the same position as an ostium secundum ASD. It is called a patent foramen ovale (PFO).[4] PFOs are distinguished by the deficiency of the septum primum. If the septum primum has developed normally, but does not fuse to the septum secundum, the defect is termed PFO.[4] There are devices available for closure of PFOs that are similar to ASD closure devices; however, this article reviews only the devices for ASD closure.

CLINICAL PRESENTATION

The clinical presentation of patients with ASDs includes normal to slightly increased precordial activity; a systolic ejection murmur; a split, second heart sound that does not vary with respiration; and, occasionally, a diastolic murmur or rumble.[4,5] The ECG of an individual with ASD may exhibit a normal sinus rhythm with right ventricular hypertrophy.[5] The chest radiograph may show evidence of a normal heart size to mild cardiomegaly, which is related to the dilated right atrium and right ventricle; increased pulmonary vascular markings with prominent pulmonary artery segments may also be evident on the chest radiograph.[5] Diagnosis of an ASD can usually be confirmed by transthoracic echocardiography. Echocardiography may show the actual defect, estimate its size, show the presence of an intracardiac shunt, and/or evaluate the connection of the pulmonary veins. Cardiac catheterization is only indicated in cases of an inconclusive echocardiographic examination or the presence of associated anomalies that may require further evaluation.

TREATMENT OPTIONS FOR ASD
Spontaneous Closure

Patients with an isolated secundum ASD and without symptoms can be monitored regularly by their cardiologists. The smaller the defect and the younger the age of the patient at diagnosis, the more likely there will be spontaneous closure of this type of ASD.[6] Sinus venosus, coronary sinus, and primum defects do not close spontaneously. Because of the posterior location of sinus venosus defects and the associated partial anomalous pulmonary venous return, surgical closure remains the treatment of choice for these types of ASD. Coronary sinus defects cannot be closed with a device because of their location. Primum defects cannot be closed with a device because of their location and frequent association with 1 or more leaflets of the AV valves.

Surgical Closure

ASDs were among the first of the congenital cardiac anomalies to be corrected by surgical intervention. In 1976, King and colleagues[7] published their attempt at the first nonoperative ASD closure with a double-umbrella device. However, the size of the delivery system needed to introduce their device was 23 French and many cardiologists did not adopt this practice.[7] The primary method of treatment of closure of most ASDs has remained surgical repair until recent improvements with interventional products and smaller delivery systems brought transcatheter delivery options to the forefront.[6]

Indications for surgical closure of ASD are the same as those for transcatheter device closure.[3] These include hemodynamically significant lesions with evidence of right ventricular volume overload on echocardiography and elective closure before a child starts school.[5] Results of surgical repair of ASDs are excellent and the average hospital stay is 3 to 4 days.[8] It is reported that, with all forms of cardiac surgery, there is a small but definite risk of surgical morbidity (5%).[9]

Techniques for surgical closure of ASDs include direct suture repair, which is reserved for small ASDs, and the more common patch repair. The material used for patch closure of ASDs may be the patient's own pericardium, commercially available bovine pericardium, or synthetic material including Gore-Tex and Dacron.[9] The surgical approach to the ASD is dependent on its location. According to Thomson and colleagues,[9] 3 surgical approaches are available: median sternotomy, right thoracostomy, or submammary. All types of ASD may be approached adequately through a median sternotomy or right thoracotomy.[5] The submammary incision may be the most cosmetic but makes some ASDs difficult to repair.[9] The term minimally invasive surgery for repair of ASDs usually refers to repair of the defect using the same techniques as open heart surgical repair, but performing the repair through a much smaller incision.[9] Most children can successfully undergo this type of repair through a small (75–100 mm) incision in the sternum. In general, the postoperative course in the hospital is shorter, (2–3 days), because of less incisional pain and discomfort.

Regardless of the choice of incision, surgical repair of ASDs includes cardiopulmonary bypass (CPB) and myocardial ischemia.[4] The typical sequence of events for CPB involves several basics steps. The patient is anesthetized, prepared, and draped.[4] The incision is made and the pericardial sac entered. Once the pericardium is entered, preparation for CPB includes heparinization of the patient, placement of the arterial and venous cannulas, clearing them of air, and connection to the bypass pump oxygenator.[4]

To repair the defect, CPB is used either with aortic cross-clamping and cardioplegia, or with electrical fibrillation, thus stopping the heart.[5] The right atrium is then opened to allow access to the septum. One potential hazard during surgical repair is air embolism, because the left side of the heart is open to air.[4] Another hazard is the possible disruption of the conduction pathway because of the close proximity to the sinoatrial node.

Once the defect is closed, the atrial incision is closed.[4] The aortic cross-clamp is removed and patient ventilation and temperature normalization is resumed.[5] Once a stable cardiac rhythm is achieved, the patient is weaned from CPB and a single drainage tube is placed before the chest is closed.[5] Postoperative complications include chest tube drainage, effusions, postpericardiotomy syndrome, and arrhythmias.[5] After hospital discharge, recovery time is approximately 2 weeks, with an additional 8 weeks without sports activities.[2]

Successful surgical closure for ASDs are 98% to 100%.[10] The asymptomatic child with an ASD deserves close follow-up by the pediatrician and pediatric cardiologist, with constant involvement of the cardiovascular surgeon.[6] Should the patient with an ASD become symptomatic with failure to thrive, or have persistent complaints such as malaise or increased respiratory infections, early surgical intervention could be warranted.[2]

Transcatheter Device Closure

During the past 2 decades, improvements in interventional products have led interventional cardiologists to reexplore the possibility of transcatheter closure of ASDs.[11,12] The transcatheter closure technique involves implantation of 1 or more devices using cardiac catheterization methods without the need for CPB and without the need to stop the heart.[10] Appropriate patient selections for this technology has been strict and limited by guidelines from the US Food and Drug Administration (FDA).[10] Based on these guidelines, safety and efficacy of these devices is measured using data from consistent follow-up appointments for patients receiving an ASD device. Currently, these patients are followed at regular intervals of 1, 3, 6, and 12 months for the first year after the procedure.[6,10,11] If there are adverse events of any type during a device placement, the FDA currently mandates that the patient be followed for up to 5 years.[6]

Defects amenable to ASD transcatheter device therapy tend to be smaller (ie, <20–25 mm in diameter).[10] Patients with defects at the upper or lower edges of the atrial septum, such as ostium primum or sinus venosus defects, are not good candidates for this procedure because these defects usually involve other abnormalities of the heart valves, or abnormal venous drainage from the lungs.[10] Because these types of ASD usually have no chance of spontaneous closure, open heart surgery is indicated for patients with these types of ASD. Transcatheter device closure of ASDs only benefits patients with ostium secundum–type ASDs.[10,11]

At present, there are no lower age limitations that preclude device implantation.[11] However, because device sizes vary, the delivery system or sheaths used for patient access must be able to accommodate the device and implant it within the septum. These delivery systems may not be applicable for use with patients who weigh less than 8 to 10 kg.[10,11] As with surgical closure of ASDs, transcatheter device closure in pediatrics may be performed under general anesthesia. Implantation of the device is performed using confirmatory measurement by angiography and transesophageal echocardiography (TEE).[10] The patient undergoing this type of procedure is also heparinized, as is the patient undergoing surgical repair of an ASD.

The usual procedure for transcatheter device closure is similar to a standard heart cardiac catheterization. Catheters are inserted into the patient's femoral veins and artery. Routine pressure measurements and oxygen levels in all chambers of the heart are then obtained. Angiograms, using fluoroscopy, are performed to determine the size of the chambers, the size of the defect, and its location within the heart. A measuring balloon catheter is used to size the defect for the appropriate-sized device.[10]

The device is then advanced into the heart through an introducer sheath. With most of the current devices, half of the device is deployed into the left side of the atrial septum, and the second half of the device is deployed on the right side of the septum, forming a sort of sandwich over the defect.[12] Within 6 to 8 weeks, the device acts as a skeleton or framework that stimulates normal tissue to grow in and over the defect.[10] For this reason, these devices can be used in growing children; although the device itself does not grow, the tissue that covers the device does, and continues to grow as the child grows.[10] The time and degree of tissue coverage is being investigated.[10,11]

Postprocedure care for patients who have received transcatheter closure of their ASDs includes bed rest for 4 to 6 hours after the procedure and, depending on the institution, possible overnight admission to an inpatient cardiology floor. Noninvasive testing during this period includes a chest radiograph the following morning, telemetry monitoring for arrhythmias, close observation of the catheterization site, and an echo-cardiograph before discharge.[6,10] The patient may complain of a sore throat (caused by the transesophageal echo probe) and some local discomfort at the catheterization site. Potential complications following these procedures are similar to those following a cardiac catheterization: infection, bleeding, bruising, vessel trauma, perforation, arrhythmias, hypersensitivity or allergic reaction, stroke, and/or death, with the addition of potential device embolization.[6,10,11] Fluoroscopy time for this procedure ranges from 0 to 43.5 minutes, with a median of 8.7 minutes.[13] Activity restrictions usually include no contact sports for 1 month and no heavy lifting (>4.5 kg) for 1 week. Most patients return to school in 2 days to 1 week.

Transcatheter devices

Transcatheter devices are tested according to FDA guidelines. The major advantage of these devices is the noninvasive approach. In 1995, the Amplatzer septal occluder (ASO) trials, a trademark of AGA Medical, were begun in the United States. In 2001, the ASO was approved by the FDA for use in children and adults with secundum ASDs.[3,11] This device consists of wire mesh frame made of nitinol, which is a nickel/titanium alloy, molded so that there is a central waist joining the left and right atrial discs.[3,11,12] The device is sized so that the central waist completely fills or plugs the defect.[11] The frame is filled with polyester fabrics to promote thrombosis and defect closure.[11] In 2002, results from a retrospective study evaluating the cost of Amplatzer catheter closure with surgical closure were published by Kim and Hijazi.[14] They reported the mean estimated cost per case for transcatheter closure was approximately $11,540 compared with the surgical cost of $21,780.[14]

Another ASD occlusion device approved by the FDA on October 3, 2007, was the Helex Septal Occluder, a trademark of W. L. Gore, Inc.[10] This product was first made commercially available in July 1999. It also consists of a nitinol wire frame in the shape of a coil covered with Gore-Tex. Each device comes in a preassembled delivery system composed of a lock and retrieval cord. Its single nitinol wire frame allows it to configure nicely to the atrial septum.[10] Its delivery system requires that the patient's femoral vein be able to accommodate the 9-French introducer sheath (weight restriction >15 kg) and the atrial septal ratio has to be proportionate to the defect size.[10] Defects that encompass a large portion of the septum are unable to seed the device without it buttonholing through the defect.[10] The atrial septal defect must measure 15 to 20 mm or less to avoid the risk of device embolization, which makes it more suitable for use in small and medium size defects.[10] Because the Helex device received FDA approval in August 2006, experience with it is limited. The suggested retail price for each device ranges from $6000 to $9000.[10]

The ASO is the most widely used ASD closure device worldwide. Although both devices have been studied for years and shown to be safe and effective in the short term compared with surgical closure, the serious complications of erosion and cardiac perforation have been identified in long-term studies as concerns with the use of ASO.[10] No case of cardiac perforation has been reported with the Helex device, but fractures of the supporting frame have been reported in a small percentage of cases.[10,15] Studies of the cause of these complications are ongoing and involve further investigations of the variability of changes in the atrial septum during different phases of the cardiac cycle.

Efficacy

Transcatheter closure of ASDs seems to offer benefits in the short term, but long-term benefits will not be known for some time.[3,10,13] Most reviewed studies show a high success rate for device closure as defined by no residual shunt at follow-up after 3 to 12 months.[3,6,10,11,13] Patients with small residual shunts after the procedure resolved in time as endothelial tissue grew over and around the device.[10] In some patients, device closure was not feasible because of the size of the ASD or inadequate septal tissue.[10,11] Other studies reported that intracatheter difficulties resulted from positioning of the device relative to the configuration of the septal plane.[3,10,11,13]

Clinical studies indicate that good short-term results lead to long-term efficacy.[6] Evidence from long-term follow-up of patients with device closure is ongoing. Echocardiograms performed at the designated time intervals after the procedure show that right ventricular function, both systolic and diastolic, may be impaired by CPB using surgical closure, but is preserved after device closure.[16,17]

A recent study from Boston Children's Hospital analyzed echocardiograms from 34 patients who underwent device closure of ASD to investigate the immediate effects of elimination of right ventricular overload on left ventricular function.[17,18] Results indicated that, after the defect was closed, left ventricular function and end diastolic volume normalize with normalization in the left ventricular shape.[17] Left ventricular dysfunction associated with right ventricular overload is immediately reversible and is independent of heart rate and afterload in these patients.[17] These findings support the use of the transcatheter approach to ASD closure in patients with anatomically suitable defects.[16]

Of the patients who receive these devices in the United States, long-term consequences will not be known for some time. However, many European studies are ongoing and continue to report that transcatheter techniques are effective and safe for the treatment of ASD compared with the conventional surgical method.[15] Follow-up examinations as mandated by the FDA can add to the patient's medical costs.[3,6] In an article showing long-term follow-up of secundum ASDs using the ASO, the Michigan Congenital Heart Center reported that, of the 94 patients who underwent secundum ASD closure with the ASO between 1998 and 2002 and who were evaluated for a total of 120 months follow-up, the ASO continues to be a safe device.[15]

Complications

Adverse events after transcatheter device implantation include device embolization (<2%), residual shunts across the atrial septum (<4%), arrhythmias (<5%), and ASD/septal size mismatch (<5%) leading to termination of the procedure.[1-9,11] Termination of the procedure is usually necessary because placement of a device that is improperly sized to the defect can lead to the obstruction of pulmonary veins or coronary sinus or to AV valve dysfunction.[6,10,11] Malpositioning or embolization of a device can lead to the need for surgical intervention in some cases.[7,11] Other difficulties result from the inability to stabilize the device because of the absence of the aortic or posterior rim.[6,10,11]

There have been recent investigations of a possible adverse effect associated with nickel used in the devices.[3,18] One study involving the Helex device reports elective removal of the device related to possible nickel allergy.[10] Another study by Vander Pluym and Dyck[18] reported that patients receiving the Amplatzer ASD device showed no increase in blood levels of nickel. However, long-term complications of an implanted device containing a high level of nickel are not yet fully known.

Another interesting adverse effect documented by patients receiving a transcatheter ASD device includes complaints of headaches, consistent with types of migraines. These complaints have been documented in the early to midterm follow-up period.[10,11,15,19] A poster presented by Bourdages[19] at the 2002 American College of Cardiology (ACC) conference described the incidence, pattern, and risk factors of headache after transcatheter ASD Amplatzer septal occlusion. He concluded that there were no identified independent risk factors and the absence of associated neurologic symptoms and the spontaneous resolution of the headache in most cases underline the benign aspect of this situation.[20] Vander Pluym and Dyck[18] speculated that these headaches may be related to the nitinol component of the device, which may trigger histamine release from the destruction of platelets aggregated on the device.[18] In a long-term follow-up by Knepp and colleagues,[15] only 2 of 159 patients who were followed for 120 months developed migraine headache. Conversely, in the same study, 2 patients who had suffered from migraine headaches before secundum ASD closure with the ASO did not have a migraine headache during the follow-up period.[15]

Other complications unique to this technology may be the possibility of clot formation on the device itself, with the risk of clot ulceration causing stroke, or a clot into the vessels of the lung.[3,6,10,11,13] At present, these problems are addressed by administering heparin during the procedure to inhibit the coagulation system and using aspirin following the procedure.[4,6,10,13] Aspirin use is needed for 3 to 6 months after device implantation.[3,10,13] However, this varies among centers.[3,10,11,13] Before discontinuing the use of aspirin, the goal is assurance that the device is fully scarred in place and incorporated in the atrial tissue.[3,10,13] In 2003, Hausdorf and colleagues[16] reported 4 deaths caused by cardiac tamponade resulting from Amplatzer device erosion through the AV valves and heart. Hausdorf and colleagues[16] suggested that, when selecting the occluder size, the question is not only how large the defect is but also how much room is between the aorta and the interatrial groove at the end of atrial systole.[16] This group also reported that, during the TEE examination, close attention must be paid to the remaining septal tissue. Thin, aneurismal, or fragile tissue must be firmly immobilized between the 2 sides of the device, with enough remaining nonfragile tissue to support the device.[16] Fisher and colleagues[1] reported 1 death resulting from cerebral infarction in a 13-year-old girl. Although cerebral infarctions in a child of this age are considered rare, her death was attributed to the Amplatzer device that had been placed across her ASD 5 years earlier.[1]

Knepp and colleagues,[15] from the University of Michigan, reported 1 death in their follow-up series. This patient was a 2-year-old with trisomy 21. Death was related to a fatal cerebrovascular accident 18 months following device placement.[15] Autopsy findings showed a left atrial thrombus adherent to the device. Further examination revealed the device to be endothelialized, and it was not known whether this patient had a hypercoagulable state.[15] Data from all the tested devices indicated that the complication rate following transcatheter ASD occlusion is approximately 5%.[3,10] These complications include the routine risks of cardiac catheterization, such as vascular injury, particularly in cases where larger device introducer systems need to be used. Problems with blood clotting or excessive bleeding are sometimes seen, particularly in younger patients.

Costs

Device closure of ASDs has been shown to be cost-effective compared with surgical closure. Because device costs vary according to the manufacturer, there is an average cost saving of $7837 for device closure compared with surgical closure, excluding the cost of the device.[3] Equipment and procedure costs may be higher for transcatheter closure than for surgery but overall costs may be reduced by avoiding intensive care unit costs and fewer days that the patient remains in the hospital.[7] Most cost analyses do not consider the shorter recovery time and the patients' resultant return to work or school. Likewise, parents of these young patients need not take as much time off work.[3] Continued data collection and further research are needed to assess patients who receive a transcatheter ASD closure device.[3,6,10,11,13] In the short term, this procedure seems to offer benefits; however, European studies have suggested that life-long follow-up is required, as it is in all patients with CHD.[11,13]

The length of, and need for, antibiotic prophylaxis against infections in the heart vary among investigators and devices. Prophylaxis lasting from 12 months following device implantation to life-long administration is suggested; however, most centers follow the American Heart Association (AHA) recommendations.[1,13] Most patients are followed up by their cardiologist at 3 to 6 months and then for 1, 2, and 3 years following device implantation, as suggested by FDA guidelines, with variable requirements for echocardiograms, chest radiographs, and electrocardiograms. Long-term risk of a permanent prosthesis in the heart is not yet known.[6]

SUMMARY

ASDs are common congenital cardiac defects that are readily corrected through several surgical approaches. There is a subgroup of patients who are currently able to be managed with transcatheter device closure. Regardless of the mode of closure, these defects are successfully closed with low associated mortality and morbidity. Each mode of ASD closure has its own associated risks and benefits. Until recently, surgical repair was the standard treatment of choice for most ASDs. Closing ASDs using a device inserted via a catheter now offers another option for selected patients with an ostium secundum–type ASD.

Experience with transcatheter closure of ASDs is limited, with more time needed to discover all that is to be learned.[10,13] More than 15 years of clinical use has helped practitioners better understand all the conveniences and difficulties of this therapeutic approach, but the procedure is complex and will require a long learning curve.[13,16] Revisions and refinement of the devices are continuously being addressed by manufacturing companies.[16] In some centers, there is now a new form of echocardiographic guidance termed intracardiac echocardiography (ICE), which may potentially eliminate the need for general anesthesia in a significant percentage of older, cooperative patients and result in further cost savings.[3] Cost savings adjustment for the 5% failure rate with device implantation is approximately $7000.[3] This remains a substantial hospital-related cost saving compared with surgical costs.[3] In addition, the decreased time needed for recovery should be considered in this cost saving. As time progresses, systemic anticoagulation and infectious prosthetic endocardial prophylaxis should be resolved with increasing clinical experience.[6,10,13] This technology is not for everyone. However, with proper patient selection, the results of device closure of ASDs may prove to be equivalent to those results obtained through standard surgical intervention.

REFERENCES

1. Fisher G, Stieh J, Uebing A, et al. Experience with transcatheter closure of secundum atrial septal defects using the Amplatzer septal occlude: a single center study in 236 consecutive patients. Heart 2003;89:199–204.
2. McMahon CJ, Feltes TF, Fraley JK, et al. Natural history of growth of secundum atrial septal defects and implantations for transcatheter closure. Heart 2002;87: 256–9.
3. Balzer D. Transcatheter closure of intracardiac shunts. Curr Sci 2004;6:717–22.
4. Chang AC, Hanley FL, Wernovsky G. Pediatric cardiac intensive care. Philadelphia: Lippincott Williams & Wilkins; 1998.
5. Nichols DG, Cameron DE, Greeley WJ, et al. Critical heart disease in infants and children. St Louis (MO): Mosby; 1995.
6. Baskett RJ, Tancock E, Ross DB. The gold standard for atrial septal defect closure: current surgical results, with an emphasis on morbidity. Pediatr Cardiol 2003;24:444–7.
7. King TD, Thompson SL, Steiner C, et al. Secundum atrial septal defect: nonoperative closure during cardiac catheterization. JAMA 1976;235:2506–9.
8. Hughes ML, Maskell G, Goh TH, et al. Prospective comparison of costs and short-term health outcomes of surgical versus device closure of atrial septal defect in children. Heart 2002;88:67–70.
9. Thomsom JR, Aburawi EH, Watterson K, et al. Surgical and transcatheter (Amplatzer) closure of atrial septal defects: a prospective comparison of results and costs. Heart 2002;87:466–9.
10. Vincent R, Raviele A, Diehl HJ. Single-center experience with the helix septal occlude for closure of atrial septal defects in children. J Interv Cardiol 2003;16: 79–82.
11. Omeish A, Hijazi Z. Transcatheter closure of ASDs in children and adults using the Amplatzer septal occlude. J Interv Cardiol 2001;14:37–44.
12. Schrader R. Catheter closure of secundum ASD using "other" devices. J Interv Cardiol 2003;16:409–12.
13. Berger F. Transcatheter closure as standard treatment for most interatrial defects: experience in 200 patients treated with the Amplatzer septal occluder. Cardiol Young 1999;9:468–73.
14. Kim J, Hijazi Z. Clinical outcomes and costs of Amplatzer transcatheter closure as compared with surgical closure of ostium secundum atrial septal defects. Med Sci Monit 2002;8(12):787–91.
15. Knepp MD, Rocchini AP, Lloyd TR, et al. Long-term follow up of secundum atrial septal defect closure with the Amplatzer septal occluder. Congenit Heart Dis 2010;5:32–7.
16. Hausdorf G, Schneider M, Fransbach B, et al. Transcatheter closure of secundum atrial septal defects with the atrial septal defect occlusion system (ASDOS): initial experience in children. Heart 2002;7:83–8.
17. Walker RE, Moran AM, Gauvreau K, et al. Evidence of adverse ventricular interdependence in patients with atrial septal defects. Am J Cardiol 2004;93(11): 1374–7.

18. Vander Pluym C, Dyck J. Does nickel toxicity occur after placement of nitinol (nickel-titanium) devices [abstract], Cardiol Young 2001; 3rd World Congress of Pediatric Cardiology and Cardiac Surgery. Toronto, Canada.
19. Bourdages, M. Incidence of headaches after percutaneous catheter closure of ASD using the Amplatzer device. Poster presentation, American College of Cardiology. Boston (MA), 2002.

Hematopoietic Stem Cell Transplantation in Children

Julie A. Kolins, RN, BSN[a],*, Cara Zbylut, RN, BSN, CPON[a],
Susan McCollom, RN, ND, CPHON[a], Victor M. Aquino, MD[b]

KEYWORDS

- Pediatric • Hematopoietic stem cell transplant • Nursing care
- Bone marrow • HLA typing • Leukemia

Hematopoietic stem cell transplantation (HSCT) has become the standard of care for several malignant and nonmalignant hematologic disorders in children.[1] The first successful HSCT was performed in the early 1960s for a child with severe combined immunodeficiency who underwent allogeneic matched sibling HSCT without conditioning.[2] In the 1970s, patients with leukemia were cured using a combination of radiation and chemotherapy, followed by matched sibling HSCT.[3] Recent advances have included improvements in human leukocyte antigen (HLA) typing, allowance for the use of unrelated blood donors, the growth of unrelated blood donor registries, such as the National Marrow Donor Program (NMDP), and improvements in the supportive care of posttransplant patients. In the United States, the NMDP and its Be the Match Registry was established in 1987 and is one of the largest donor registries.[4] It is estimated that more than 800,000 HSCTs have been performed worldwide with a total of 55,000 to 60,000 annually.[5] Autologous and allogeneic transplants performed worldwide continue to grow at a rate of 15% to 20% per year.[5]

The outcome of HSCT in children depends on the underlying disease and remission status, the type of donor and degree of HLA match, and the health and age of the recipient.[1] The overall 5-year survival rate for children who undergo HSCT for acute myelogenous leukemia is 70%,[6,7] and 50% for those with acute lymphoblastic leukemia.[8,9] Cure rates for metastatic neuroblastoma are approaching 50% with autologous HSCT and immunotherapy with retinoic acid.[10] Children who undergo HSCT for a nonmalignancy have a survival rate of 85%.[1] Transplantation-related

The authors have nothing to disclose.
[a] Center for Cancer and Blood Disorders, Children's Medical Center, 1935 Medical District Drive, Dallas, TX 75235, USA
[b] Division of Pediatrics, Department of Pediatric Hematology/Oncology, University of Texas Southwestern Medical Center at Dallas, 5323 Harry Hines Boulevard, Dallas, TX 75390-9063, USA
* Corresponding author.
E-mail address: julie.kolins@gmail.com

mortality, defined as death caused by complications from the procedure, occurs in 5% to 10% of autologous HSCT, 10% to 20% of matched sibling allogeneic HSCT, and 20% to 40% of unrelated donor allogeneic HSCT.[1] The indications for HSCT in children with malignant and nonmalignant disorders can be found in **Box 1**. This article includes an overview of the types of HSCT, the procedures for collection of stem cells, HSCT environmental considerations, the HSCT process, potential acute and chronic complications, and specialized HSCT nursing care.

HSCT TYPES

Hematopoietic stem cells (HSC) are pluripotent, immature cells that differentiate into cells that produce the different components of the blood[11] (ie, red blood cells [RBC], white blood cells [WBC], and platelets). HSCs are harvested from a donor (either the recipient [autologous] or another person [allogeneic]) and infused into the recipient to restore normal hematopoietic function. Donor selection is based on the underlying diagnosis and remission status of the HSCT recipient. Bone marrow, peripheral blood, and umbilical cord blood (UCB) are 3 potential sources of HSC. In

---

Box 1
Selected indications for HSCT in children with malignant and nonmalignant disorders

Malignant disorders

Acute lymphoblastic leukemia

    First remission: hypodiploidy, induction failure

    Second remission: early relapse (<36 months from complete remission), late relapse

    Third or greater remission

Acute myelogenous leukemia

    First remission: Flt-3 mutation, monosomy 5 or 7, induction failure

    Second or greater remission

Juvenile myelomonocytic leukemia

Myelodysplastic syndrome

Chronic myelogenous leukemia: refractory or relapse after tyrosine kinase therapy

Neuroblastoma

Recurrent brain tumors (eg, medulloblastoma)

Recurrent Hodgkin lymphoma

Recurrent non-Hodgkin lymphoma

Recurrent germ cell tumors

Nonmalignant disorders

Aplastic anemia

Fanconi anemia

β-Thalassemia

Sickle cell anemia

Primary immunodeficiency disorders (eg, severe combined immunodeficiency, Wiskott-Aldrich syndrome)

Inborn errors of metabolism (eg, Hurler syndrome, Hunter syndrome)

the future, if bioengineering of embryonic stem cells comes to fruition, the current methods of HSCT may change. As previously mentioned, there are currently 2 types of HSCT autologous and allogeneic.

Autologous

An autologous transplant involves HSC collection from the recipient. The only contra-indication to autologous collection is the presence of malignant cells in the bone marrow of the recipient because of the risk of host tumor contamination. Autologous HSCT is not performed in children with nonmalignancies because they have a genetic defect in their HSC.[12] Peripheral blood stem cells are the preferred source for autolo-gous transplant because of their more rapid hematopoietic reconstitution after trans-plantation compared with other stem cell sources.[1,13] The advantages of autologous transplant include convenient access to the HSC, fewer infectious complications because of more rapid WBC engraftment, and no risk of graft-versus-host disease (GVHD) from donor T lymphocytes.[1] However, most patients with relapsed leukemia who receive an autologous HSCT have an increased risk of another relapse because of the absence of a graft-versus-leukemia (GVL) effect from donor T lymphocytes.[1] Several cancers and other diseases are commonly treated with autologous HSCT, such as acute myelogenous leukemia and autoimmune disorders.[1] Autologous HSCT is a treatment choice for certain pediatric solid tumors, such as high-risk neuro-blastoma and high-risk Ewing sarcoma.[13,14]

Allogeneic

Allogeneic HSCT requires HSC from a donor other than the recipient. Several cancers and anemias are commonly treated with allogeneic HSCT, such as acute myeloge-nous leukemia, acute lymphoblastic leukemia, and aplastic anemia.[1] Allogeneic HSCT is rarely a treatment option for pediatric solid tumors because of high risks for GVHD and other complications.[14]

HLA are surface antigens whose genes are found on chromosome 6 of human cells.[1] These antigens make up the major histocompatibility complex, which allow T lymphocytes to detect foreign cells.[1] Each parent contributes 1 set of HLA antigens and alleles, making the probability of perfectly matching a sibling approximately 25%.[1] There is an antigen and allele pair for each HLA set. An ideal HSCT donor has HLA-A, HLA-B, HLA-C, and HLA-DRB1 antigens and alleles identified and matched using high-resolution typing for a total of 8 matched alleles.[15,16] The importance of other HLA antigens and alleles, such as DQB1 and DPB1, is not fully understood; however, DQB1, along with HLA-A, HLA-B, HLA-C, and HLA-DRB1, is commonly analyzed in donors for a full match of 10 alleles.[15,17]

Although an identical twin would be a complete match to the recipient's HLA (ie, syngeneic HSCT), the lack of GVL makes the use of this donor source in leukemias less appealing.[1] Therefore, a matched sibling related donor with an 8/8 or 10/10 HLA match is the donor source of choice for allogeneic HSCT.[17] The use of a sibling or rela-tive with a single mismatch has shown equivalent survival rates compared with a completely matched family donor, albeit with a higher risk of GVHD.[18] In the absence of a family donor, a matched unrelated donor is sought. There is an approximate 80% probability of finding an HLA-A, HLA-B, and HLA-DRB1 matched unrelated donor via the NMDP.[19] Adult donors who are complete or 1 antigen mismatched can be selected; however, there is an unacceptably high risk of severe GVHD or death asso-ciated with 2 or more antigen mismatches.[1]

Allogeneic transplants may use HSC obtained from peripheral blood, bone marrow, or UCB. Transplantation with allogeneic peripheral blood stem cells is associated with an increased risk of chronic GVHD compared with bone marrow stem cell transplantation because of higher T lymphocyte numbers from the donor.[1,13] Allogeneic HSCT using UCB units allows for a greater degree of HLA mismatch because the risk for GVHD is lower[1,13,16]; however, UCB units contain less HSC per unit compared with bone marrow and peripheral blood HSC units.[15]

COLLECTION OF HSCs

Bone marrow and peripheral blood HSC donation is a detailed and controlled process whereby healthy stem cells are obtained. The volunteer HSC donor age range is 18 to 60 years for the Be the Match Registry.[4] A thorough HSC donor evaluation includes a physical examination, a complete history to rule out genetic diseases, a urinalysis, laboratory testing (eg, complete blood count with differential, chemistry profile, coagulation screen, infectious disease testing, crossmatching, and confirming HLA typing), a chest radiograph, and a pregnancy test if applicable.[20] The sources from which HSC are collected are described later.

Bone Marrow Stem Cell Collection

Bone marrow is harvested from the donor's posterior or anterior iliac crests.[1] The procedure is usually performed in a hospital operating room under general or local anesthesia.[1] The risks to the donor are minimal and include pain at the biopsy site, anesthesia side effects, fatigue, and headache.[1,21]

Peripheral Blood Stem Cell Collection

To obtain an adequate amount of peripheral blood stem cells, bone marrow–suppressive chemotherapy and/or granulocyte colony-stimulating factor (G-CSF) are common agents given to the donor before leukapheresis.[1] G-CSF, such as filgrastim (Neupogen), stimulates the proliferation and mobilization of HSC from the bone marrow.[1] Leukapheresis is the process of separating WBC from blood circulation and returning the remainder of the blood to the donor's circulation.[22] An automated machine collects the donor's HSC for about 4 to 6 hours through peripheral or central venous catheters,[1,22] while the remaining cells are reinfused into the donor. The donated cells are mixed in heparin, acid-citrate dextrose A, and preservatives (eg, dimethyl sulfoxide [DMSO]) and then cryopreserved.[22] The benefit of peripheral collection for the donor is avoidance of general anesthesia. Risks to the donor involve hypocalcemia (eg, paresthesia) from the acid-citrate dextrose A anticoagulation preservative[23] and side effects from G-CSF, such as bone pain and headache.[22] There may also be complications from the placement of large-bore intravenous (IV) catheters or femoral central venous catheters.[22]

UCB Stem Cell Collection

UCB is a third source for stem cells. An advantage of UCB stem cells is easy collection immediately after birth with no risk to the donor.[1,24] Infectious disease testing of the mother's blood is done during the collection period.[25] The HSC are cryopreserved in a cryomedium, such as DMSO, at a UCB bank.[26] UCB stem cells have less risk for GVHD and a decreased chance of viral disease transmission for the transplant recipient.[24] Because of rapid availability, allowance for HLA mismatch, and other benefits, UCB stem cells are becoming an attractive transplant option.[1,13]

ENVIRONMENTAL CONSIDERATIONS FOR HSCT

There are no established national standards defining the environmental requirements of an HSCT unit.[27] However, the Centers for Disease Control and Prevention (CDC), along with 2 other organizations, developed evidence-based guidelines for infection prevention in patients receiving blood and marrow stem cell transplants who received myeloablative therapy (ie, full-dose conditioning of the patient's bone marrow before HSC infusion).[28] The following are highly recommended guidelines based on efficacy and improvement in overall survival.[28] Strict adherence to standard contact precautions is important when vancomycin-resistant enterococci[27] and/or *Clostridium difficile* is present in a patient.[28] Health care workers with diseases transmissible by air, droplet, or direct contact (eg, varicella zoster virus, infectious gastroenteritis, herpes simplex virus (HSV) lesions of lips or fingers, and upper respiratory tract infections) should not provide care for a patient receiving HSCT.[28] In addition, visitors with communicable illnesses should not enter an HSCT unit.

There are no conclusive data to confirm whether the following infection control practices should be the standard of care for HSCT.[27] Most HSCT centers have private patient rooms, high-efficiency particulate air (HEPA) filtration, controlled room ventilation with positive air pressure, correctly sealed rooms, and high rates of room air exchange.[28] Other infection control measures may include strict visitor screening policies; restricted bathroom sharing; isolation and barrier precautions (eg, N95 respirators during patient transport); limited dust and fungi in the HSCT recipient's environment (eg, recipient avoidance of construction areas); diet restrictions (eg, raw seafood, eggs, blue cheese, fresh fruits and vegetables); controlled, clean water; 2 sets of HSCT unit entrance double doors to reduce exposure to air contaminated with fungal spores; infection control surveillance; strict equipment management; and prohibition of fresh flowers or live plants.[27]

In an HSCT unit, proper equipment for emergency care must always be accessible. Cardiorespiratory and pulse oximetry monitors, oxygen, and suction equipment should be readily available in the patient's room as well. Some hospitals have designed outpatient HSCT facilities based on an extensive evaluation of risks versus benefits and a thorough psychosocial and economic assessment of the HSCT recipient.[29] Although partial and complete autologous and allogeneic HSCT have been performed in an outpatient setting, currently there are not enough data to confirm the safety of outpatient allogeneic HSCT.[27] In contrast, outpatient autologous HSCT can be safely performed, especially when peripheral blood stem cells are used,[30] recipients receive reduced-intensity conditioning regimens,[1] and frequent follow-up can be assured. Outpatient HSCT is increasing in popularity, in part because of reports stating that there is comparable patient safety with significant potential cost reduction.[30]

THE PROCESS OF HEMATOPOIETIC STEM CELL TRANSPLANT

HSCT consists of 3 phases[1]: a pretransplant phase (ie, conditioning),[2] infusion of HSC, and[3] a posttransplant phase, during which engraftment occurs and hematopoietic function is restored. Survival rates and the incidence of complications vary depending on the donor and recipient ages, the recipient's underlying diagnosis, and the health of the recipient at the time of transplantation.[13]

Pretransplant Phase

The underlying diagnosis, remission status, and health of the recipient are the most important factors when selecting the type of transplant and conditioning regimen.[31] Once the decision is made to proceed to transplant, the recipient undergoes a more extensive evaluation. The evaluation consists of organ function tests, such as a chest radiograph, an echocardiogram or multigated acquisition scan for left ventricular ejection fraction measurement, an electrocardiogram, pulmonary function testing, an I-125 Glofil glomerular filtration rate or creatinine clearance test, an audiogram, and an ophthalmic examination.[31] Dental examination, dietary assessment, and neuropsychological testing are performed. Numerous laboratory studies including liver function tests, infectious disease tests, serum immunology studies, thyroid function tests, coagulation screens, crossmatching, and HLA reconfirmation are performed.[31] Diagnostic scans, bone marrow biopsies, and lumbar punctures are performed depending on the underlying disease.[31] The recipient's functional status is assessed (eg, using a Karnofsky or Lansky performance score), and the recipient's comorbidity index is determined by the transplant coordinators using a model specifically for this purpose.[31] When applicable, sperm banking and egg harvesting for the HSCT recipient are discussed with the patient and family.[1]

Before HSCT, the type and timing of conditioning and preparative regimens vary depending on the recipient's disease state, remission status, previous complications, type of donor HSC, and institutional expertise. The purpose of conditioning is to suppress the recipient's immune system to prevent graft rejection (eg, allogeneic HSCT), eradicate any malignant cells, and create space for the recipient's new bone marrow.[1] Generally, total-body irradiation (TBI), high-dose chemotherapy, and immunosuppressive agents (**Table 1**) are given 4 to 9 days before the stem cell infusion.[32] Myeloablative conditioning regimens completely destroy the existing bone marrow and suppress the recipient's immune system to prevent rejection of the donor graft[1] (ie, the recipient's hematopoietic recovery only occurs with the donor HSCs).[14] Nonmyeloablative regimens have less toxic adverse effects and less bone marrow suppression but still allow for HSC engraftment in the recipient's bone marrow.[1] The preparative days also commonly include supportive therapies, such as IV fluid hydration, anticonvulsants, IV protective agents (eg, mesna), corticosteroids, antipyretics, and antihistamines, as well as the frequent monitoring of blood and urine testing to assess organ function.[32] See **Table 2** for selected myeloablative and nonmyeloablative agents used for HSCT.

Table 1 Selected pediatric HSCT immunosuppressive agents for GVHD prevention and treatment	
Agent/Treatment	**Notable Adverse Effects**
Antithymocyte globulin (ATGAM)	Fever, chills, hypotension, rash, anaphylaxis
Corticosteroids	Mood swings, hypertension, hyperglycemia, gastrointestinal bleeding, osteoporosis, cushingoid syndrome
Cyclosporine (Sandimmune)	Nephrotoxicity, hypertension, magnesium wasting, hyperkalemia, tremors, seizures
Methotrexate (Mexate)	Nephrotoxicity, hepatotoxicity, mucositis
Mycophenolate mofetil (Cellcept)	Abdominal pain, vomiting, hypertension, nephrotoxicity
Sirolimus (Rapamune)	Hypertension, diarrhea, peripheral edema, rash
Tacrolimus (Prograf)	Nephrotoxicity, hypertension, magnesium wasting, hyperkalemia, tremors, seizures
Thalidomide (Synovir)	Peripheral neuropathies, constipation, sedation, teratogenic effects

Data from Kline NE, editor. Essentials of pediatric hematology/oncology nursing: a core curriculum. 3rd edition. Glenview (IL): Association of Pediatric Hematology/Oncology Nurses; 2008. p. 106.

Table 2
Selected pediatric HSCT myeloablative and nonmyeloablative conditioning agents

Agent	Notable Side Effects	Notable Nursing Implications
TBI	Bone marrow suppression, gastrointestinal mucositis, altered skin integrity	Narcotics, antiemetics, good oral care
Cyclophosphamide (Cytoxan)	Nausea, vomiting, syndrome of inappropriate antidiuretic hormone, hemorrhagic cystitis	Antiemetics, serum electrolyte levels, urine testing for blood, IV hydration fluids and mesna, voiding often and good urinary output
Etoposide (Toposar)	Nausea, vomiting, hypotension	Antiemetics
Busulfan (Myleran)	Seizures	Frequent busulfan pharmacokinetic levels with the first dose to prevent toxicity, prophylactic anticonvulsants
Fludarabine (Fludara)	Nausea, vomiting, mucositis	Antiemetics
Melphalan (Alkeran)	Vesicant, nausea, vomiting	Antiemetics, good urinary output (IV hydration fluids, furosemide), short drug stability
Thiotepa (Thioplex)	Integumentary excretion causes irritation, mucositis	Frequent skin care (baths, new linens, loose clothing, no occlusive dressings), use a filter with administration, dilute with normal saline before use, avoid direct contact with patient
Carboplatin (Paraplatin)	Electrolyte imbalance, delayed nausea and vomiting	Antiemetics, avoid drug-aluminum contact, audiology examinations
Cisplatin (Platinol)	Electrolyte imbalance, delayed nausea and vomiting, nephrotoxicity, ototoxicity	Magnesium sulfate, calcium gluconate, and/or mannitol IV hydration fluids, antiemetics, avoid drug-aluminum contact, maintain good urinary output, audiology examinations
Carmustine (BCNU)	Late pulmonary dysfunction, nausea, vomiting, marked facial flushing	Use glass containers and polyethylene-lined administration sets for stability, protect from light, antiemetics
Cytarabine (Cytosar-U)	Nausea, vomiting, flulike symptoms, conjunctivitis, mucositis	Antiemetics, steroid eye drops

Abbreviation: BCNU, 1,3-*bis*(2-chloroethyl)-1-nitrosourea.

Data from Kline NE, editor. The pediatric chemotherapy and biotherapy curriculum. 2nd edition. Glenview (IL): Association of Pediatric Hematology/Oncology Nurses; 2007. p. 17, 18, 41, 42, 44–46, 49, 54.

Hematopoietic Stem Cell Infusion

The day of HSC infusion (day 0) is anticlimactic but a happy day for the patient and the patient's caregivers. Sometimes it is referred to as a patient's second birthday. Central IV access should be in place before HSCT conditioning begins. A long-term central venous catheter[33] or implanted vascular access device (IVAD)[34] is required for HSCT because of the numerous medications, supportive IV therapies, and blood products the patient will receive, as well as serving as an access for blood specimens. The donor HSC units may be RBC or volume reduced depending on the recipient's ABO type and the volume to be infused. HSC are never irradiated or filtered, unlike other blood products.[33]

Frozen HSC are normally infused for autologous HSCT and HSC units are thawed in a hot water bath before infusion. After transfusion, the DMSO preservative from the HSC unit(s) is excreted through the recipient's pulmonary system for 1 to 2 days, causing a bad taste in the mouth and a strong malodorous smell.[35] Adverse effects of DMSO include nausea, vomiting, abdominal cramping, flushing of the skin, transient cardiac arrhythmias, renal failure, and anaphylaxis.[36,37] Before, during, and after the rapid gravity IV infusion of stem cells, cardiac monitoring, pulse oximetry, and vital sign trending are recommended.[32] Other potential adverse effects from frozen HSC include hypertension, hemoglobinuria, micropulmonary emboli, fluid overload, and infection.[31]

Prehydration fluids may be necessary 4 to 12 hours before the infusion of frozen cells.[32] Shortly before the HSC infusion, the nurse should be prepared to premedicate the patient with 1 or more of the following: an antihistamine, antipyretic, antiemetic, and/or corticosteroid. After the infusion, the nurse may administer posthydration fluids for 12 to 24 hours and diuretics to maintain renal perfusion.[32] Careful intake and output measurements are priorities for 12 to 24 hours after HSC infusion.[32]

Unpreserved (fresh) stem cells are normally used for allogeneic HSCT. Fresh HSC look similar to platelet or packed RBC units, depending on RBC depletion. The infusion is commonly given over 1 to 4 hours to prevent fluid overload. If there is ABO incompatibility, hemolysis and hematuria are expected after the recipient receives the HSC infusion. Potential adverse effects from fresh cells include anaphylaxis, hypertension, hemolytic transfusion reactions, micropulmonary emboli, and infection.[31]

The nurse administering fresh stem cells should be prepared to administer premedications, such as antihistamines, antipyretics, corticosteroids, and diuretics. Prehydration fluids may be necessary for 12 to 24 hours before the HSC infusion if there is ABO incompatibility and/or the patient has had a prior transfusion reaction.[1] Posthydration fluids may be given as well.[32] Commonly, a minimum of 2 mL/kg/h of urine output is necessary for 12 to 24 hours after the infusion.[32,38]

Posttransplant Phase

Engraftment
Engraftment is the process by which HSC enter the recipient's body and resume making WBCs, RBCs, and platelets. The first 100 days are considered a waiting period while the newly infused stem cells begin to function and produce the vital components of blood. During the engraftment phase, production of WBCs occurs first, followed by RBCs, and finally platelets. Engraftment is usually defined by the number of neutrophils and platelets detected on the peripheral blood smear.[1] The absolute neutrophil count (ANC) is calculated by the following formula: total WBC count multiplied by the sum of the percentage of segmented neutrophils and number of bands.[32] WBC engraftment is defined as an ANC greater than 500/mm^3 for 3 consecutive days or a single ANC greater than 1500/mm^3.[3,32] Platelet engraftment is defined as having a platelet count of greater than 20,000/mm^3 and not supported by a platelet transfusion in the previous 7 days.[32] If the donor and HSCT recipient are of a different blood type, the recipient's blood type will change with time. In general, WBC engraftment occurs 7 to 14 days after peripheral blood stem cell infusion, 10 to 21 days after bone marrow stem cell infusion, and 10 to 28 days after UCB stem cell infusion.[39]

The timing of engraftment is variable and dependent on a variety of factors. The primary factor in the rapidity of engraftment is the HSC source and number of cells infused.[1] The rate of engraftment is fastest when peripheral blood cells are infused and slowest when UCB cells are used.[1] In general, engraftment after autologous HSCT is more rapid than allogeneic HSCT.[1]

Nursing implications, discharge planning, and follow-up

The nursing care from day 0 to discharge focuses on the prevention and management of expected and unexpected complications and toxicities. The HSCT nurse must have excellent time management and prioritization skills to administer numerous HSCT-related medications, manage high-acuity patients, and coordinate care with other disciplines.

Multidisciplinary teamwork is imperative to enhance communication and coordination in the pediatric HSCT setting (Box 2). Multidisciplinary teamwork increases quality of care, addresses medical and psychosocial aspects of care, and improves collaboration.[40] Teamwork promotes the development of innovative ideas and solutions for complex patient issues.[40] Daily rounding on an HSCT unit with the primary health care providers is a means to promote effective team communication.[41] Institutions also use care conferences when there are complex physical and psychosocial problems associated with patients having HSCT.

Discharge planning begins on admission and continues throughout the HSCT process. After engraftment is complete, discharge teaching becomes a primary focus

---

Box 2
Common services represented in the HSCT multidisciplinary team

Medical providers: Attending, Fellow, Advanced Practice Nurse/Physician Assistant, Resident/Intern

Consultations with specialists (eg, cardiologist, nephrologist)

Inpatient HSCT nurses

Patient and his/her caregivers

Pharmacist

Respiratory therapist

Registered dietician

Medical social worker

Outpatient HSCT nurses

Clinical psychologist

Case manager/family educator

Physical, occupational, speech, and massage therapists

Child life specialist

Music therapist

Patient care assistant

Transplant coordinator

School reintegration coordinator

Housekeeping

Health Unit Coordinator

Chaplin

in the patient's plan of care. Usually, patients require an additional 2 to 3 weeks to recover from the nonhematopoietic toxicities of the conditioning, such as mucositis and diarrhea. In general, children are required to be afebrile, able to take oral medications, and to be sufficiently mobile to maintain a daily schedule before being discharged. Before discharge, the home is prepared by cleaning the air ducts and carpets if present. For the first 100 days, it is strongly recommended that pets, especially cats, birds, and reptiles, live outside the home, and potted plants are removed from the house.[32] A low-bacteria diet is recommended, including avoidance of restaurant food and certain raw foods. Caregiver education must be completed and skills documented before discharge (eg, central line care and knowledge of medication schedule). It is important for the nursing staff to educate patients and caregivers about potential complications at home (eg, fever, prolonged bleeding, severe vomiting or diarrhea, level of consciousness changes, breathing difficulties, rashes, central line exudate, weight loss, headaches, coughing, or fatigue). Patients are then seen frequently in the outpatient setting (ie, normally 2 to 3 times per week in the immediate discharge period), and then less frequently as they improve clinically.[32]

HSCT recipients maintain central venous access devices for extended periods of time while being treated at the transplant center and after the initial discharge; however, the length of time is variable and individualized.[33] For example, regardless of RBC, WBC, and/or platelet engraftment, the HSCT recipient may continue to be blood product transfusion–dependent even after discharge from the HSCT center.[42] In addition, the recipient may continue to receive IV outpatient prophylaxis, such as IV immunoglobulin (IVIG).[43] Moreover, if the recipient develops GVHD or the underlying disease relapses or reoccurs and central venous access is necessary, the original central venous access device may be used.

POTENTIAL ACUTE COMPLICATIONS OF HEMATOPOIETIC STEM CELL TRANSPLANTATION

Bone Marrow Suppression (Neutropenia, Anemia, and Thrombocytopenia)

Seven to 10 days after transplant conditioning begins, all cell lines in the bone marrow will be absent.[32] Until the donor's stem cells engraft in the recipient's bone marrow, there are inadequate WBC, RBC/hemoglobin, and platelet levels. Commonly, a complete blood count with differential will be evaluated frequently for the patient receiving HSCT.

Neutropenia

A decreased WBC count, or leukopenia, creates a risk for common and opportunistic infections, especially when the ANC is less than 500/mm^3.[32] Environmental infection control measures,[28] hand washing, clean or sterile technique for nursing and medical care, excellent central line care, meticulous body hygiene, and medication prophylaxis are important.[32] Invasive equipment, such as urinary catheters and nasogastric tubes, should not be inserted into body orifices unless the benefits outweigh the risks. Careful nursing assessments should include a thorough inspection for infection. Although patients with an infection may have a fever, cough, sore throat, rectal pain, dysuria, erythema, edema, or exudate present, a neutropenic patient may not exhibit a typical response to an infection; the only presenting sign may be a fever.[32]

Anemia

Anemia ranges from a hemoglobin less than 13.5 g/dL in newborn infants to less than 12.0 g/dL in children 12 to 16 years of age.[43] Common signs and symptoms of anemia are tachycardia, pallor, fatigue, shortness of breath, and dizziness.[43] Packed RBC transfusions are commonly administered when the hemoglobin is less than 8 g/dL or the HSCT recipient is symptomatic.[32] Institutional policy dictates standard packed RBC dosing and infusion rates, but the dose and rate may be reduced depending on the patient's individual clinical status. Respiratory compromise may be seen in patients with a hemoglobin less than 7 g/dL, and oxygen therapy and/or other medical support may be necessary.

Thrombocytopenia

A decreased platelet count, or thrombocytopenia, is defined as a platelet count less than 50,000/mm³.[32] Platelet transfusions are given when the platelet level falls to less than 10,000/mm³ to 20,000/mm³ or if the patient is actively bleeding.[32] Patients having HSCT may have epistaxis, gingival or oral mucosa bleeding, prolonged clotting times, headaches, dizziness, vision changes, blood-tinged sputum, hematuria, hematemesis, hematochezia, ecchymosis, or petechiae.[43] The risks versus benefits of jet-injector medications, needle blood samples, IVAD accessing, and intramuscular injections should be assessed in patients with thrombocytopenia. Patients should be encouraged to use soft toothbrushes, avoid constipation, never use suppositories, enemas, or rectal thermometers, avoid excessive pressure when voiding or blowing their noses, take oral steroids with food, and avoid medications with ibuprofen and acetylsalicylic acid.[32]

Infections

Bacterial, viral, and fungal pathogens are common causes of infection in HSCT recipients. Bacterial infection is a common cause of septic shock and often the need for intensive care support in children undergoing HSCT is high.[44] As a result of the conditioning regimen, the patient develops pancytopenia lasting from 2 to 4 weeks, which leads to a profound immunodeficiency state and extremely high susceptibility to opportunistic infections. After engraftment, neutrophil and lymphocyte dysfunction can lead to an increased risk of infection for up to 1 year after transplantation, or beyond if chronic GVHD is present. Toxicities of the preparative regimen, such as skin breakdown and mucositis, increase the risk of septicemia caused by bacteremia with oral, skin, and gastrointestinal (GI) flora.[45] In allogeneic HSCT recipients, GVHD and the need for immunosuppressive therapy contribute to the development of infection.

Prophylactic interventions

A variety of agents are used to prevent infection in HSCT recipients (**Table 3**). Good hand washing is the most effective way to prevent infections.[28] Viral screening for cytomegalovirus (CMV), Epstein-Barr virus (EBV), adenovirus, and other viral agents may be performed weekly via polymerase chain reaction (PCR) tests. Although serum galactomannan and Beta-D-glucan can be used as a screening test for fungal infection, the diagnostic usefulness of these tests in pediatric patients is associated with a false-positive rate when compared with adults and is not accurate in patients receiving piperacillin/tazobactam (Zosyn).[46] Despite the use of prophylactic agents, the prompt initiation of antibiotics at the time of fever, and/or evidence of infection and supportive care in the intensive care setting, the risk of death from infection in the first 100 days after HSCT is 5% to 10%.[44]

Timing of infections

The timing of infections is related to the stage of hematopoietic recovery following transplantation and is divided into early, middle, and late phases.[44] HSCT nurses can use their knowledge of blood cell line recovery during these phases to anticipate potential complications and intervene as early as possible.

Table 3
Selected prophylactic agents used in the prevention of infections in pediatric HSCT recipients

Agent	Infection Prevented
Acyclovir	HSV
Acyclovir, valacyclovir, ganciclovir, foscarnet	CMV-positive patients or donors
Fluconazole	Candida species
Voriconazole, itraconazole, liposomal amphotericin B, caspofungin	Candida, Aspergillus
Bactrim, pentamidine, dapsone	Pneumocystis jiroveci (formerly Pneumocystis carinii)
Levaquin, ciprofloxacin, other antibiotics	Bacterial infection
IVIG	Viral, bacterial infection
G-CSF	Bacterial, fungal infection

Abbreviation: CMV, cytomegalovirus.

The early phase is defined as the first 29 days after transplantation, in which there is severe neutropenia. Patients are at the highest risk of infection during this time. The most common pathogens are gram-negative bacilli (eg, Enterobacter sp, Escherichia coli, Klebsiella, and Pseudomonas) and gram-positive cocci (eg, streptococci, staphylococci, and enterococci).[47] Fungal infections with Candida may occur secondary to mucositis.

The middle phase is defined as day 30 to 100 after transplantation, when engraftment has occurred, but immune cell function has not returned to normal. The risk for bacterial infection is less; however, infections with CMV, EBV, and adenovirus are encountered, as well as fungal infection with Candida and mold infection, such as Aspergillus species.[48]

The late phase is defined as the period after day 100 after HSCT. In the absence of GVHD, the risk of infection is fairly low. Immune dysfunction seen during this time is related to the development of chronic GVHD and its treatment. Patients are at risk for pneumococcal infection because of splenic dysfunction,[49] viral, and fungal infections.

Recognition of infection and treatment
Nursing assessment of the HSCT recipient is critical in the successful prevention and management of infection. With the development of an initial fever (defined as a temperature of 38.5°C once or 2 or more temperatures of 38°C in a 24-hour period),[32] the patient should be assessed for signs and symptoms of infection, and blood and other cultures (eg, urine, cerebrospinal fluid) should be obtained.[32] Broad-spectrum antibiotics should be administered immediately and vital signs monitored closely for signs of septic shock and need for intensive care support. Vancomycin combined with a third-generation cephalosporin or antipseudomonal penicillin, based on institutional bacterial sensitivity monitoring, should be started immediately and is potentially lifesaving.[44] Anaerobic coverage may be added in the presence of severe mucositis, diarrhea, or evidence of perianal infection.[44] Aminoglycoside therapy should be added if the patient has clinical or laboratory evidence of septic shock or in patients with gram-negative bacteremia[44]; serum aminoglycoside levels are commonly monitored to prevent toxicity. Other antibiotics may be administered based on the identification of infectious agents and their antibiotic sensitivity profile.

If fever persists for more than 4 days and no source of infection can be determined, an undiagnosed fungal infection should be suspected. Day 5 of continual fevers tends to be a busy day for the nurse and patient because some centers perform an endoscopic nasal examination, a computed tomography (CT) scan of the chest, and an abdominal ultrasound to assess for fungal disease.[32] Empiric fungal therapy, such as liposomal amphotericin B or caspofungin, should be administered. Amphotericin B and its less toxic derivatives have severe adverse effects, such as fever, chills, hypotension, nephrotoxicity, hepatotoxicity, hypokalemia, and hypomagnesemia.[38] The patient may have a biopsy of any suspicious lesions to direct antimicrobial therapy. If radiographic or clinical evidence of a pneumatic process is present, bronchoalveolar lavage or open lung biopsy should be considered and galactomannan assays sent on the fluid.[50] If esophagitis is suspected, endoscopy should be performed to rule out candidal or HSV esophagitis. Diarrhea may be evaluated with stool cultures and colonoscopy. Multiple episodes of positive blood cultures may require removal of the patient's central venous catheter.

Reactivation and infection with CMV is a common occurrence.[51] In the preantiviral era, the mortality from CMV in the posttransplantation period was 25%.[51] Ganciclovir prophylaxis for CMV is effective in preventing and treating CMV; however, the development of neutropenia associated with the drug can lead to bacterial and fungal infections.[38] The development of PCR-based blood testing for CMV has led to the practice of weekly monitoring of CMV and use of ganciclovir for treatment if reactivation occurs.[52] If a patient develops ganciclovir-resistant CMV or cannot tolerate therapy because of severe neutropenia, foscarnet or cidofovir can be given as alternative therapy based on the HSCT center's CMV prophylaxis policies.

GI Toxicity

Nausea, emesis, and diarrhea can be bothersome for the HSCT recipient when other complications are also occurring. However, nausea, emesis, and diarrhea may begin during initiation of the preparative regimen and continue into the first couple of weeks after the HSC infusion.[32] Numerous factors contribute to continued nausea and vomiting, such as medications, infections, GVHD, or slow mucosal healing. Diarrhea beyond this period may be caused by medication(s), infection, refeeding syndrome, or GVHD. The nurse should assess for signs and symptoms of abdominal discomfort, dehydration, electrolyte imbalance, and integumentary irritation. The nurse can help significantly decrease the patient's severity of GI issues by anticipating potential nausea and vomiting and diligently assessing antiemetic effectiveness and the need for breakthrough antiemetic management (**Table 4**). A barrier cream may be helpful for skin breakdown caused by episodes of diarrhea.

Mucositis from myeloablative conditioning and immunosuppressive agents (eg, methotrexate) may begin by the third day after the HSC infusion and peak by the seventh to 10th day.[1,32] Mucositis may occur anywhere along the GI tract, presenting as painful ulcerations. Ulcer healing may begin by the 12th day, often coinciding with WBC engraftment. Diligent pain management with IV opioids may be necessary, and a patient-controlled analgesia pump is sometimes needed for severe pain. Parenteral nutrition is administered when weight loss occurs from excessive oropharyngeal and GI mucositis.[1] Anorexia may start during conditioning and extend for several months after the transplant.[32] A change in taste sensation, xerostomia, damaged mucosa, nausea and vomiting from the transplant process, and GVHD are some of the common causes of anorexia.[1,32]

High-quality nursing assessments of the GI system are imperative to diagnosing altered integrity of the GI tract. Common nursing care for GI complications is to weigh the patient at least once a day in the morning and assess intake and output measurements at least every 2 to 4 hours. The nurse should also give scheduled antiemetic agents

Table 4
Selected antiemetic medications for pediatric HSCT recipients

Medication	Class	Purpose
Ondansetron (Zofran), granisetron (Kytril)	Serotonin receptor antagonist	Prophylaxis of nausea and vomiting: preparative regimen
Dexamethasone (Decadron)	Corticosteroid	Breakthrough or prophylaxis of nausea and vomiting: preparative regimen
Lorazepam (Ativan): adjunct use	Benzodiazepine	Breakthrough of nausea and vomiting: after HSC infusion
Aprepitant (Emend)	Neurokinin-1 receptor antagonist	Prophylaxis of delayed nausea and vomiting: preparative regimen
Promethazine (Phenergan): not first line, Chlorpromazine (Thorazine), Prochlorperazine (Compazine)	Phenothiazine	Breakthrough of nausea and vomiting: preparative regimen, after HSC infusion
Diphenhydramine (Benadryl): adjunct use	Antihistamine	Breakthrough of nausea and vomiting: preparative regimen
Haloperidol (Haldol): not first line	Dopamine antagonist and butyrophenone	Breakthrough or refractory nausea and vomiting
Metoclopramide: not first line	Dopamine antagonist	Prophylaxis of refractory nausea and vomiting
Dronabinol (Marinol): not first line	Cannabinoid	Prophylaxis of refractory nausea and vomiting

Data from Chemotherapy and radiotherapy treatment guidelines for nausea and vomiting micromedex 2.0, (electronic version). Greenwood Village (CO): Thomson Reuters (Healthcare). Available at: http://www.thomsonha.com. Accessed November 26, 2010.

and assess the need for antiemetics as needed (see **Table 4**), as well as administer IV fluids, nasogastric tube feedings, total parenteral nutrition, and fat emulsion.[32] Stool cultures and/or occult blood tests may be necessary for patients with diarrhea. The nurse should encourage good oral, skin, and perineal hygiene. Some patients may benefit from a dietary consult with a registered dietician for an individualized nutrition plan.

Hyperengraftment Syndrome (Capillary Leak Syndrome)

During the neutrophil recovery phase, patients may experience symptoms of hyperengraftment syndrome regardless of transplant type. Symptoms may include a skin rash, fever (with no identifiable infectious cause), hypoxia, pulmonary infiltrates, and hepatic and renal insufficiencies.[53–55] The cause is not completely understood but is believed to be the result of an interaction between cytokines released during neutrophil recovery causing inflammation and capillary injury.[56,57] The capillaries may become diffusely permeable (capillary leak), which clinically manifests as edema, ascites, effusions, and weight gain.[56,58]

Although these symptoms are typically self-limited, supportive therapy is usually necessary. Nursing care includes symptom relief by administering antipyretics for fevers, oxygen for hypoxia, diuretics for weight gain, edema, ascites, and effusions, and a renal dose of dopamine. Because of the patient's neutropenic status, a fever should always be investigated for an infectious cause. Applicable interventions include obtaining blood cultures from all available lumens, administration of antibiotics, antivirals, and antifungals, as well as other tests (eg, chest radiograph, ultrasound of the abdomen, and CT scan of the chest). If these tests are negative and there seems to be no infectious cause, corticosteroids are the standard treatment of engraftment syndrome and capillary leak. The threshold for initiating steroid therapy depends on center expertise. Steroid initiation is beneficial because of the immunosuppressive effect on the cytokine reactions and its anti-inflammatory nature.[56,59] Symptoms typically resolve once engraftment has occurred.

Veno-Occlusive Disease

Veno-occlusive disease (VOD) is an inflammatory condition in the liver that causes narrowing or occlusion of the small veins, resulting in obstruction and/or reversal of blood flow.[60,61] Risk factors for VOD include preexisting liver dysfunction, advanced disease status at the time of transplantation, greater HLA mismatch between donor and recipient, and intense conditioning regimens. VOD usually occurs within the third to fourth week after transplantation.[60–62]

The diagnosis of VOD is essentially a combination of clinical symptoms including hepatomegaly, right upper quadrant pain, ascites, sudden weight gain, hyperbilirubinemia, jaundice, and altered coagulopathy.[58,61] Increased liver function tests, altered coagulation studies, severe thrombocytopenia, and hypoalbuminemia are associated abnormal laboratory values.[62] In addition, a liver ultrasound with a Doppler ultrasound study will likely be performed to confirm obstruction or reversal of blood flow. This complication is typically self-limiting in children; however, the severity and mortality associated with VOD increase the importance of prophylactic therapy. Prophylactic therapies include alprostadil (prostaglandin E1), ursodiol (Actigall), pentoxifylline (Pentopak), continuous heparin infusions, and low-molecular-weight heparin.[61,63–65] Defibrotide is effective in the treatment of VOD; however, it is currently available only on a compassionate-use basis in the United States.[61,66–68]

The nursing role in managing patients with VOD is aimed at reducing the fluid accumulation, controlling the pain, and correcting the coagulopathy. Therefore, patients will likely be using patient-controlled analgesia for pain, as well as receiving multiple transfusions of blood products. Nurses need to be aware of the complications associated with narcotic use, be competent in blood product administration, and administer diuretics as indicated. Additional assessments are intake, output, abdominal girths, weight measurement, coagulation studies, and liver and kidney function studies.

Graft Failure

Definitions and causes

Graft failure is defined as the lack of hematopoietic function following autologous or allogeneic HSCT.[1] Failure to achieve sustained engraftment is associated with significant morbidity and mortality (eg, infection, bleeding, and/or relapse of the patient's primary disease). Graft failure can be caused by immunologic rejection of the graft in allogeneic HSCT recipients or by the infusion of inadequate numbers of HSC (see **Table 5** for causes of graft failure). Graft failure can be divided into primary (early) and secondary (late) graft failure. Primary graft failure is manifested by the failure to achieve an ANC of greater than 500 cells/mm^3 by day 28 after transplantation.[69,70] Secondary graft failure is defined by loss of previously achieved graft function as shown by lack of production of 2 hematopoietic cell lines.[39] Poor graft function is manifested as failure to achieve adequate blood counts following allogeneic HSCT in the presence of complete donor engraftment. Incomplete donor engraftment can occur with evidence of donor and recipient engraftment (mixed chimerism).[71] The incidence of graft failure varies and is dependent on the underlying disease and donor source. It is estimated that the risk of graft failure after an autologous HSCT is 1% to 5% and

Table 5
Selected causes of graft failure in pediatric HSCT recipients

Cause	Rationale
Patients with aplastic anemia or β-thalassemia who receive more than 40 RBC transfusions	Production of recipient antibodies to donor HLA antigens
Reduced-intensity conditioning regimens	Insufficient immunosuppression to allow engraftment
UCB units for HSCT	Less total HSC infused compared to peripheral blood and bone marrow stem cells infused
Pretreatment with chemotherapy	Graft manipulation
Increase in the number of HLA mismatches	Production of recipient antibodies to donor HLA antigens
Advanced donor and recipient age	Production of recipient antibodies to donor HLA antigens
Infection with viruses (eg, CMV, EBV, adenovirus, parvovirus B19, human herpesvirus 6, human herpesvirus 8)	Viral suppression of bone marrow function
Relapse of the underlying disease	Replacement of donor cells with non functioning malignant ones

Data from Refs.[32,39,104]

5% to 20% after an allogeneic HSCT; it is highest with an unrelated HSCT donor.[1] In general, patients who undergo transplantation for a nonmalignancy have a higher risk of graft failure than those with an underlying malignancy.

Diagnosis and treatment

If graft failure occurs, patients should be screened for infectious causes and a bone marrow aspiration and biopsy should be performed to assess for evidence of engraftment or recurrence of the recipient's underlying disease. Viral infections should be aggressively treated with IVIG and antiviral agents. If malignancy recurs, withdrawal of immunosuppression or donor lymphocyte infusion could be attempted to induce a GVL effect. Several strategies may be used in the management of graft failure. Increasing the patient's immunosuppressive therapy may reverse graft failure and may lead to restoration of immune function. Growth factors, such as G-CSF or erythropoietin, may allow for an increase in blood counts and reduce the risk of infection in patients with poor engraftment. Infusion of donor lymphocytes or CD34+ stem cells may reverse graft failure.[1] A second transplant either from the original donor or another donor with a second conditioning regimen may be necessary to correct graft failure.

Nursing implications

Patients are monitored with daily complete blood count with differential studies during the engraftment phase to assess for signs of graft failure.[32] Nursing assessments to detect signs of infection, such as fever, tachycardia, and poor perfusion, could potentially be lifesaving. Patients should also be assessed for signs of easy bruising, bleeding, and/or pallor, which could be signs of thrombocytopenia or anemia.

Acute GVHD

Acute GVHD occurs when T lymphocytes from the donor attack the recipient's various tissue antigens. The inflammatory response and cytokine release kill recipient cells and disrupts tissues. The sites most often affected by acute GVHD are the skin, liver, and gut.[60,72] Acute GVHD usually occurs in the first 2 to 5 weeks after transplant. Skin GVHD presents as an erythematous, maculopapular rash, beginning on the palms and soles, but it can be diffuse in nature. Additional involvement is shown by generalized erythroderma, with possible bullous formation and desquamation.[60] Liver GVHD manifests in the form of increased liver enzymes and varying levels of hyperbilirubinemia. When GVHD occurs in the gut, patients have watery green diarrhea, abdominal pain, decreased appetite, and anorexia, often accompanied by bleeding and persistent nausea and vomiting.[60] Because of the potential mortality of acute GVHD, most efforts are focused on prevention, early detection, and treatment. Commonly used immunosuppressive agents for GVHD prophylaxis and treatment are listed in **Table 1**. For acute GVHD occurrences, corticosteroids are the most commonly used first-line agent.[60,72]

Nursing considerations for acute GVHD include recognizing the early warning signs, including subtle skin rashes and generalized pain, right upper quadrant pain, diffuse abdominal pain, sudden changes in nausea/vomiting, and increased diarrhea.[1] Strict monitoring of the patient's intake and output and fluid and electrolyte statuses are important nursing implications. Aggressive antiemetic therapy and pain medications may be indicated for patient comfort. Stool replacement therapy in extreme cases may be necessary for hemodynamic stability. The nurse should prepare patients for skin or rectal biopsies and endoscopy procedures if ordered. Nursing interventions for acute GVHD of the skin include hypoallergenic moisturizers and gel or porcine dressings.[32]

Pulmonary Complications

Pulmonary complications are classified as infectious or noninfectious and early or late. The risks of the complication are related to the underlying disease, conditioning regimen, type of HSCT, and the presence of GVHD. Pulmonary complications occur in 30% to 60% of HSCT recipients[73]; however, morbidity and mortality are reduced the earlier the complication is diagnosed and treated.[74] Rapid assessment of changes in baseline pulmonary status and diagnosis using sputum cultures, CMV tests, bronchoalveolar lavage, and lung biopsies may be potentially lifesaving.

Pulmonary edema

During the early part of the posttransplant phase, increased capillary permeability is common because of large volumes of fluid as well as renal and cardiac dysfunction secondary to HSCT-related agents. Other causes include TBI, sepsis, and immunosuppressive agents.[74] Clinical manifestations from fluid in the lungs include dyspnea, weight gain, crackles, hypoxemia, and possible cardiomegaly.[38] Aggressive use of diuretics is a common treatment, and intubation in an intensive care setting may be necessary if the edema cannot be controlled.

Radiation pneumonitis

Patients receiving HSCT who receive TBI as part of their conditioning regimen have a 7% risk of developing radiation pneumonitis (ie, inflammation of the lungs).[75] The risks for radiation pneumonitis are dose of radiation, amount of tissue affected, and any preexisting lung disease. Common clinical manifestations are dyspnea, cough, and fever; however, often it is an incidental finding from a chest radiograph.[75] Increased lactate dehydrogenase and C-reactive protein are 2 common laboratory findings. Development of radiation pneumonitis can occur from 1 to 3 months after radiation.[75] Pulmonary function testing in patients with radiation pneumonitis reveals restrictive lung physiology and reduced diffusion lung capacity. The primary treatment of symptomatic patients is corticosteroids with a gradual wean.[75]

Interstitial pneumonitis

Interstitial pneumonitis/pneumonia secondary to infection from bacteria, fungi, or viruses is associated with high rates of morbidity and mortality[73]; however, mortality is low with bacterial pneumonitis caused by broad-spectrum antibiotic usage. Different causes are associated with the different stages of hematopoietic recovery following HSCT: the early phase, the middle phase, and the late phase. The early phase is associated with bacterial (eg, gram-negative) and candida infections caused by neutropenia and altered mucocutaneous integrity.[74] If neutropenia persists, aspergillus becomes a concern. In the middle phase of impaired cell-mediated immunity, CMV, pneumocystis, and aspergillus are the predominate pathogens causing infectious pulmonary complications.[73,76] In the late phase, allogeneic HSCT recipients have poor cell-mediated and humoral immunity and are more susceptible to CMV, varicella, and EBV infections.[73]

Fungus-related infections often have a mortality rate as high as 90%.[73,74] Aspergillus is typically acquired through inhalation; therefore, environmental control measures are important to help prevent this complication.[28] The clinical symptoms of aspergillus are nonspecific and include fever, productive cough, and pleuritic pain. Radiographic imaging typically shows nodules and diffuse infiltrates, with late diagnosis associated with cavitations. The halo sign is a common feature seen with radiography. Because of the high mortality associated with fungal infections, the use of empiric therapy is common. Common first-line therapy is voriconazole and amphotericin B or its derivatives as an adjunct. The length of the therapy varies with extent of infection, response, and correction of the underlying immune deficit.[73]

CMV is the most common viral pathogen causing lower respiratory tract infection and is the major viral infection causing death in HSCT recipients.[73] CMV pneumonitis may occur 6 to 12 weeks after HSCT.[74] Most of the general population has been exposed to CMV, which results in the potential for active disease caused by reactivation of the latent virus. Patients commonly experience low-grade fever, nonproductive cough, tachypnea, and hypoxemia during virus reactivation.[73,74]

A variety of methods are used to diagnose CMV pneumonitis. Chest radiograph and/or CT scan show patchy or diffuse ground-glass opacities with pulmonary nodules. In addition, CMV PCR can be used to test blood, urine, and respiratory secretions. The most definitive method of diagnosis is bronchoalveolar lavage fluid. The use of CMV seronegative blood products and CMV prophylactic medications, such as acyclovir, ganciclovir, and foscarnet, has helped reduce the occurrence of CMV infections.[73] The primary treatment of active CMV infection is high-dose IVIG and ganciclovir, foscarnet, or cidofovir; however, all of these medications may cause bone marrow and organ toxicities. Close monitoring of laboratory tests is necessary when treating patients with CMV infections. However, even with current treatment options, the mortality is 50% once a patient develops clinical symptoms of CMV pneumonitis.[73] Currently, researchers are trying to develop a CMV vaccine; however, development has been a challenge, as new strains of CMV continue to evolve.[77]

Alveolar hemorrhage

A serious but uncommon complication is diffuse alveolar hemorrhage. This clinical syndrome begins with injury to the alveolar capillaries, arterioles, and venules and leads to RBC accumulation in the distal air spaces. The cause is unknown; however, one possibility is the influx of neutrophils and cytokines into the lungs, because the complication occurs 7 to 21 days after HSCT during the engraftment period.[32] Clinical signs and symptoms are dyspnea, nonproductive cough, hypoxia, fever, increasing blood seen on successive aliquots of bronchoalveolar lavage fluid, and the absence of an infectious cause from fluid cultures. Chest radiography is often nonspecific, making it difficult to distinguish the adverse effect from other pulmonary complications. Definitive diagnosis is bronchoalveolar lavage with diffusely hemorrhagic fluid. Regardless of early diagnosis and treatment with platelet transfusions, high-dose corticosteroids, and mechanical ventilation in an intensive care setting, alveolar hemorrhage is associated with a high inpatient mortality.[74,75]

Nursing implications

Nursing interventions consist of measures to help detect pulmonary complications and support the potentially life-threatening sequelae. Blood gas specimens, blood products, supplemental oxygen, and ventilation may be necessary in an intensive care setting.[32] Close attention to pulse oximetry trends, oxygen requirements, and fever is critical in monitoring patients receiving HSCT. The nurse should help or encourage the patient to follow strict institutional mouth care and skin care regimens to decrease early bacterial infections related to mucosal breakdown that could lead to pulmonary complications. Supporting and maintaining the appropriate environmental controls decreases the patient's risk for acquiring a fungal infection.[28] The nurse should educate patients and caregivers regarding the purpose and importance of medications, such as antiviral therapies and steroids, and therapies.[32]

Renal Complications

Because of the basic functions of toxin filtration, waste excretion, and fluid and electrolyte maintenance, the kidneys are highly susceptible to damage during the HSCT process. Various nephrotoxic agents are used during the conditioning and posttransplant phases. These agents are responsible for most acute renal failures in patients receiving HSCT, as well as other complications, including sepsis, GVHD, and VOD.[78–80] Decreased blood flow is another cause of acute renal failure. Kidney damage causes improper filtering of electrolytes, proteins, and glucose, resulting in proteinuria, electrolyte imbalances, and increased blood urea nitrogen and creatinine levels.[60] Nursing considerations for patients with acute renal failure should focus on the early warning signs, such as hypertension, hematuria, proteinuria, and electrolyte imbalances (eg, hyperkalemia), as well as supportive care associated with these symptoms. Common nursing implications are measuring body weight and monitoring intake and output as ordered. Medication levels of nephrotoxic medications (eg, cyclosporine, vancomycin, amphotericin B) should be monitored per institutional policy. Impaired renal function in an HSCT recipient may require diuretics, antihypertensives, and/or reduced medication dosing. More severe cases of renal dysfunction may require a renal dose of dopamine, renal replacement therapy, or continuous venovenous hemofiltration.

Hemorrhagic cystitis is defined as painful hematuria secondary to inflammation of urinary bladder epithelial cells.[81] Early onset hemorrhagic cystitis can be attributed to damage inflicted by drugs used during conditioning, such as a metabolite of cyclophosphamide.[82–84] Preventative therapy includes adequate hydration, frequent urination, and mesna in conjunction with cyclophosphamide. Viral infections causing damage to the urinary bladder, such as *Polyomavirus hominis* type 1 (BK virus), *Polyomavirus hominis* type 2 (JC virus), and adenovirus, are late in onset and often are more severe in nature.[84–86] Clinical manifestations of hemorrhagic cystitis include gross hematuria and dysuria, decreased hemoglobin levels in severe cases, large clots in the bladder, and urinary obstruction. An ultrasound may be used to visualize clots.[83] Nursing assessments include strict intake and output measurement, urine testing, urine cultures, and assessment for urinary pain. Treatment of hemorrhagic cystitis is limited and focuses on vigorous hydration, antiviral therapy if a virus is detected, continuous bladder irrigation for severe cases, and cystoscopy.[81] Nursing considerations include maintaining hydration, transfusing blood products, and managing pain with medications.

LATE EFFECTS OF HSCT

Improvements in supportive care have led to improved survival rates for children undergoing HSCT. However, an increasing incidence of long-term complications is being recognized. In a recent study by Bhatia and colleagues,[87] patients who underwent an HSCT had a tenfold increased risk of experiencing a late mortality compared with the general population. Eighteen percent of HSCT recipients who were disease free 2 years after transplantation died because of late complications.[87] A large number of patients experience long-term chronic complications, and 19% reported a problem that prevented them from going to work or attending school.[87] Common late effects of HSCT include chronic GVHD, immunosuppression, endocrine dysfunction, posterior cataracts, pulmonary complications, secondary malignancies (eg, leukemias and solid tumors), and disease relapse.[32]

Endocrine Dysfunction

Endocrine dysfunction is common in HSCT survivors.[88] Thyroid, pituitary, and gonadal dysfunction are seen, especially in children who received TBI during conditioning. Reduced fertility and sterility seem to be common in HSCT recipients.[89,90] Recent studies have shown a decrease in the number of children born to survivors of HSCT compared with their siblings. Children and adolescents also experience growth failure, which is related to the development of chronic GVHD and the use of radiation therapy.[91,92] Growth failure may be caused by growth hormone deficiency syndrome or a wasting syndrome associated with chronic GVHD. Survivors should be screened with appropriate tests of thyroid and gonadal function and monitored closely for growth failure. Sperm banking and embryo cryopreservation should be considered in appropriate candidates before transplantation.[1] However, ova cryopreservation is not currently available in most centers.

Selected Late Complications Requiring Hospitalization

HSCT recipients may be hospitalized for the following late complications: immunosuppression and infection (eg, varicella zoster, CMV, pneumocystis pneumonia, adenovirus, parainfluenza virus), chronic GVHD, respiratory compromise (eg, interstitial pneumonitis, restrictive disease, obstructive disease), active bleeding (eg, esophageal strictures), uncontrolled hypertension, vomiting, diarrhea, dehydration, and altered mental status or seizures.[1,32]

Chronic GVHD disease

Chronic GVHD has a significant negative impact on the quality of life of long-term survivors of HSCT and is the most common cause of morbidity and mortality after HSCT.[93–95] Chronic GVHD is a chronic autoimmune disease and often resembles collagen vascular disease seen in adults. Patients with chronic GVHD commonly present with sicca syndrome (eg, dry, burning, itching eyes), xerostomia, oral ulcerations, changes in taste, and skin changes (eg, dyspigmentation, desquamation, lichenoid changes).[32] Other organs involved include the GI tract (eg, esophageal strictures, malabsorption), liver (eg, increased liver function, cholestasis), lungs, and vaginal mucosa.[32] The patient may have scleroderma, short stature, failure to thrive, hair loss, brittle nails, weight loss, contractures, and generalized immunosuppression. Treatment consists of prolonged steroid and other immunosuppressive therapies (eg, cyclosporine, tacrolimus) (see **Table 1**). Patients with chronic GVHD are at high risk for infection and should be admitted to the hospital if fever occurs or the patient seems clinically ill.

Pulmonary dysfunction
Diffuse lung damage remains a significant problem after transplantation and can occur in 25% to 55% of HSCT recipients.[76,96,97] Cytotoxic agents (eg, busulfan), TBI, infectious pathogens, and chronic GVHD are risk factors for the development of pulmonary dysfunction after HSCT.[32] HSCT recipients are monitored yearly with pulmonary function testing to allow for early detection of pulmonary dysfunction. The treatment of patients who develop chronic lung disease is corticosteroid therapy and antibiotics if infection is present.

Noninfectious bronchiolitis obliterans typically occurs 6 to 12 months after HSCT, and rarely occurs in autologous HSCT recipients. Bronchiolitis obliterans is characterized by inflammation of the small airways and nonreversible airflow obstruction. The cause is unclear, but there is evidence that it is related to bronchial mucosal damage caused by GVHD.[73,76] Presenting symptoms are dry cough, dyspnea, and fever.[73] The best method for diagnosis is surgical lung biopsy. The primary treatment is corticosteroids with response to therapy within 1 to 3 months.[73] There is no effective medical treatment except the use of high-dose steroids. The mortality is more than 65% within 3 years of HSCT.[74,75]

Secondary malignancies
Survivors of HSCT have an increased risk of cancer compared with the general population.[98,99] Risk factors for the development of secondary malignancies include the use of TBI, the development of chronic GVHD, and T lymphocyte depletion of the graft before HSCT. In general, secondary leukemias occur earlier (within the first 2 years), and solid tumors occur later. The estimated annual incidence of secondary malignancy in HSCT survivors is 3.5% at 10 years and 12.8% at 15 years after allogeneic HSCT.[98,99]

Disease recurrence
Relapse of the primary disease is still the most common cause of death in children who undergo HSCT for malignancy.[100] The risk of relapse is related to the type of cancer, the remission status of the patient, and the number of remissions the patient had before HSCT.[32] The chance of survival for patients who relapse after HSCT remains poor. Treatment options include a second HSCT, donor lymphocyte infusions, or further conventional chemotherapy.

SPECIALIZED NURSING CARE FOR HEMATOPOIETIC STEM CELL TRANSPLANT PATIENTS

The medical management and nursing care of patients receiving HSCT are highly specialized and complex. Although the CDC provides guidelines for infection prevention and treatment[28] and the Foundation for the Accreditation of Cellular Therapy (FACT) has established international standards for cellular therapy centers,[101] there are no standardized protocols or guidelines for nursing care. Many standards of practice originate from professional organizations, such as the Association of Pediatric Hematology/Oncology Nurses[102]; however, many HSCT centers are requesting evidence-based practice guidelines for establishing nationwide standard nursing practice.

As more institutions achieve FACT accreditation, the standards and policies for the care of patients receiving HSCT are becoming more universal. Nursing education must focus on understanding preparative regimens, supportive care, posttransplant complications, infections, and toxicities. The comprehension of complex pharmacology management is imperative to excellent HSCT nursing care. Having strength in these areas allows the nurse to better understand HSCT, to better care for the patients, and to better educate the patients' caregivers.[32]

Although the stress experienced by the family cannot be matched, being an HSCT nurse has its own stressors. These nurses help provide treatments causing morbidity and mortality. Medical treatments and the applicable nursing interventions may worsen current conditions or cause the patient to exchange one disease for another (eg, the patient's leukemia may be cured after HSCT, but now he/she lives with chronic GVHD). HSCT nurses are expected to detect subtle changes at the bedside and often have standing orders allowing for independent decisions.[103] Pediatric HSCT challenges the nurse's knowledge and skill set; however, HSCT nursing offers satisfaction and hope when patients overcome their complex complications requiring hospitalization and are competent to leave the transplant center and start the next phase in their HSCT journey.

SUMMARY

The medical management and nursing care of the HSCT recipient are complex because of the extensive pathophysiology and process of HSCT, numerous medications and therapies required for HSCT, acute and chronic complications, adverse effects, resources involved, various environmental considerations, and potential for morbidity and/or mortality. The HSCT process and therapies may affect any body system, requiring proficient and prioritized nursing care. Knowledge and competence in the pre-HSCT conditioning regimens, the process of HSC infusion, the high-acuity care of patients after HSCT, and the timing of potential adverse effects and complications are necessary to care for the complex HSCT recipient. Although autogenic and allogeneic HSCT are curative treatment options, there are risks for morbidity and/or mortality, and HSCT recipients may be readmitted for hospitalization at any time after HSCT.

REFERENCES

1. Copelan EA. Hematopoietic stem-cell transplantation. N Engl J Med 2006;354: 1813–26.
2. Gatti RA, Meuwissen HJ, Allen HD, et al. Immunological reconstitution of sex-linked lymphopenic immunological deficiency. Lancet 1968;2:1366–9.
3. Thomas ED, Buckner CD, Banaji M, et al. One hundred patients with acute leukemia treated by chemotherapy, total body irradiation, and allogeneic marrow transplantation. Blood 1977;49:511–33.
4. Who We Are - About the National Marrow Donor Program. National Marrow Donor Program Web site, 2010. Available at: http://www.marrow.org/ABOUT/Who_We_Are/index.html. Accessed February 17, 2011.
5. Horowitz MM. Uses and growth of hematopoietic cell transplantation. In: Appelbaum FR, Forman SJ, Negrin RS, et al, editors, Thomas' hematopoietic cell transplantation, vol. 4. Oxford (UK): John Wiley and Sons; 2008. p. 15–21.
6. Rubnitz JE. Childhood acute myeloid leukemia. Curr Treat Options Oncol 2008; 9:95–105.
7. Sisler IY, Koehler E, Koyama T, et al. Impact of conditioning regimen in allogeneic hematopoetic stem cell transplantation for children with acute

myelogenous leukemia beyond first complete remission: a pediatric blood and marrow transplant consortium (PBMTC) study. Biol Blood Marrow Transplant 2009;15:1620–7.

8. Pui CH, Evans WE. Treatment of acute lymphoblastic leukemia. N Engl J Med 2006;354:166–78.

9. Smith AR, Baker KS, Defor TE, et al. Hematopoietic cell transplantation for children with acute lymphoblastic leukemia in second complete remission: similar outcomes in recipients of unrelated marrow and umbilical cord blood versus marrow from HLA matched sibling donors. Biol Blood Marrow Transplant 2009;15:1086–93.

10. Matthay KK, Villablanca JG, Seeger RC, et al. Treatment of high-risk neuroblastoma with intensive chemotherapy, radiotherapy, autologous bone marrow transplantation, and 13-cis-retinoic acid. N Engl J Med 1999;341:1165–73.

11. Weissman IL. Stem cells: units of development, units of regeneration and units in evolution. Cell 2000;100:157–68.

12. Biffi A, Cesani M. Human hematopoietic stem cells in gene therapy: pre-clinical and clinical issues. Curr Gene Ther 2008;8(2):135–46.

13. Ljungman P, Urbano-Ispizua A, Cavazzana-Calvo M, et al. Allogeneic and autologous transplantation for haematological diseases, solid tumours and immune disorders: definitions and current practice in Europe. Bone Marrow Transplant 2006;37:439–49.

14. Barrett D, Fish JD, Grupp SA. Autologous and allogeneic cellular therapies for high-risk pediatric solid tumors. Pediatr Clin North Am 2010;57(1):47–66.

15. Rocha V, Gluckman E; Eurocord-Netcord registry and European Blood and Marrow Transplant group. Improving outcomes of cord blood transplantation: HLA matching, cell dose and other graft- and transplantation-related factors. Br J Haematol 2009;147:262–74.

16. Shaw BE, Arguello R, Garcia-Sepulveda CA, et al. The impact of HLA genotyping on survival following unrelated donor haematopoietic stem cell transplantation. Br J Haematol 2010;150:251–8.

17. Shaw BE, Mayor NP, Russell NH, et al. Diverging effects of HLA-DPB1 matching status on outcome following unrelated donor transplantation depending on disease stage and the degree of matching for other HLA alleles. Leukemia 2010;24(1):58–65.

18. Hough R, Cooper N, Veys P. Allogenic haemopoietic stem cell transplantation in children: what alternative donor should we choose when no matched sibling is available? Br J Haematol 2009;147(5):593–613.

19. Dahlke J, Kröger N, Zabelina T, et al. Comparable results in patients with acute lymphoblastic leukemia after related and unrelated stem cell transplantation. Bone Marrow Transplant 2006;37(2):155–63.

20. Horowitz MM, Confer DL. Evaluation of hematopoietic stem cell donors. Hematology Am Soc Hematol Educ Program 2005;469–75.

21. Körbling M, Anderlini P. Peripheral blood stem cell versus bone marrow allotransplantation: does the source of hematopoietic stem cells matter? Blood 2001;98(10):2900–8.

22. Hölig K, Kramer M, Kroschinsky F, et al. Safety and efficacy of hematopoietic stem cell collection from mobilized peripheral blood in unrelated volunteers: 12 years of single-center experience in 3928 donors. Blood 2009;114(18):3757–63.

23. Adamski J, Griffin AC, Eisenmann C, et al. Increased risk of citrate reactions in patients with multiple myeloma during peripheral blood stem cell leukapheresis. J Clin Apher 2010;25(4):188–94.

24. Locatelli F. Improving cord blood transplantation in children. Br J Haematol 2009;147:217–26.
25. Weinberg A, Enomoto L, Li S, et al. Risk of transmission of herpesviruses through cord blood transplantation. Biol Blood Marrow Transplant 2005;11(1): 35–8.
26. Son JH, Heo YJ, Park MY, et al. Optimization of cryopreservation condition for hematopoietic stem cells from umbilical cord blood. Cryobiology 2010;60(3): 287–92.
27. Hayes-Lattin B, Leis JF, Maziarz RT. Isolation in the allogeneic transplant environment: how protective is it? Bone Marrow Transplant 2005;36(5):373–81.
28. Sullivan KM, Dykewicz CA, Longworth DL, et al. Preventing opportunistic infections after hematopoietic stem cell transplantation: the Centers for Disease Control and Prevention, Infectious Diseases Society of America, and American Society for Blood and Marrow Transplantation Practice Guidelines and beyond. Hematology Am Soc Hematol Educ Program 2001;392–421.
29. McDiarmid S, Hutton B, Atkins H, et al. Performing allogeneic and autologous hematopoietic SCT in the outpatient setting: effects on infectious complications and early transplant outcomes. Bone Marrow Transplant 2010;45:1220–6.
30. Gonzalez–Ryan L, Haut PR, Coyne K, et al. Developing a pediatric outpatient transplantation program: The Children's Memorial Hospital experience. Front Biosci 2001;6:G1–5.
31. Hamadani M, Craig M, Awan FT, et al. How we approach patient evaluation for hematopoietic stem cell transplantation. Bone Marrow Transplant 2010;45: 1259–68.
32. Kline NE, editor. Essentials of pediatric hematology/oncology nursing: a core curriculum. 3rd edition. Glenview (IL): Association of Pediatric Hematology/ Oncology Nurses; 2008. p. 98–108.
33. Sovinz P, Urban C, Lackner H, et al. Tunneled femoral central venous catheters in children with cancer. Pediatrics 2001;107(6):E104.
34. Kim HJ, Yun J, Kim HJ. Safety and effectiveness of central venous catheterization in patients with cancer: prospective observational study. J Korean Med Sci 2010;25(12):1748–53.
35. Santos NC, Figueira-Coelho J, Martins-Silva J, et al. Multidisciplinary utilization of dimethyl sulfoxide: pharmacological, cellular, and molecular aspects. Biochem Pharmacol 2003;65(7):1035–41.
36. Del Mastro L, Venturini M, Viscoli C, et al. Intensified chemotherapy supported by DMSO-free peripheral blood progenitor cells in breast cancer patients. Ann Oncol 2001;12(4):505–8.
37. Davis JM, Rowley SD, Braine HG, et al. Clinical toxicity of cryopreserved bone marrow graft infusion. Blood 1990;75(3):781–6.
38. Bakitas Whedon M, Wujcik D, editors. Blood and marrow stem cell transplantation: principles, practice and nursing insights. 2nd edition. Sudbury (MA): Jones and Bartlett; 1997. p. 17–8, 168, 299.
39. Baron F, Baker JE, Storb R, et al. Kinetics of engraftment in patients with hematologic malignancies given allogeneic hematopoietic cell transplantation after nonmyeloablative conditioning. Blood 2004;104:2254–62.
40. Patel DR, Pratt HD, Patel ND. Team processes and team care for children with developmental disabilities. Pediatr Clin North Am 2008;55(6):1375–90.
41. Mittal VS, Sigrest T, Ottolini MC, et al. Family-centered rounds on pediatric wards: a PRIS network survey of US and Canadian hospitalists. Pediatrics 2010;126(1):37–43.

42. Sariosmanoglu N, Uğurlu B, Turgut NH, et al. Use of tunnelled catheters in hae-matological malignancy patients with neutropenia. J Int Med Res 2008;36(5): 1103–11.
43. Schmidt-Hieber M, Schwarck S, Stroux A, et al. Prophylactic i.v. Igs in patients with a high risk for CMV after allo-SCT. Bone Marrow Transplant 2009;44(3): 185–92.
44. Ninin E, Milpied N, Moreau P, et al. Longitudinal study of bacterial, viral, and fungal infections in adult recipients of bone marrow transplants. Clin Infect Dis 2001;33:41–7.
45. Ruescher TJ, Sodeifi A, Scrivani SJ, et al. The impact of mucositis on alpha-hemolytic streptococcal infection in patients undergoing autologous bone marrow transplantation for haematologic malignancies. Cancer 1998;82:2275–81.
46. Lau A, Chen S, Sleiman S, et al. Current status and future perspectives on molecular and serological methods in diagnostic mycology. Future Microbiol 2009;4:1185–222.
47. Collin BA, Leather HL, Wingard JR, et al. Evolution, incidence, and susceptibility of bacterial bloodstream isolates from 519 bone marrow transplant patients. Clin Infect Dis 2001;33:947–53.
48. Marr K, Boeckh AM, Carter RA, et al. Combination antifungal therapy for inva-sive aspergillosis. Clin Infect Dis 2004;39:797–802.
49. Haddad PA, Repka TL, Weisdorf DJ. Penicillin-resistant *Streptococcus pneumo-niae* septic shock and meningitis complicating chronic graft versus host disease: a case report and review of the literature. Am J Med 2002;113:152–5.
50. Bergeron A, Belle A, Sulahian A, et al. Contribution of galactomannan antigen detection in BAL to the diagnosis of invasive pulmonary aspergillosis in patients with hematologic malignancies. Chest 2010;137(2):410–5.
51. Bueno J, Ramil C, Green M. Current management strategies for the prevention and treatment of cytomegalovirus infection in pediatric transplant recipients. Paediatr Drugs 2002;4(5):279–90.
52. Ghaffari SH, Obeidi N, Dehghan M, et al. Monitoring of cytomegalovirus reacti-vation in bone marrow transplant recipients by real-time PCR. Pathol Oncol Res 2008;14:399–409.
53. Madero L, Vicent MG, Sevilla J, et al. Engraftment syndrome in children under-going autologous peripheral blood progenitor cell transplantation. Bone Marrow Transplant 2002;30:355–8.
54. Edenfield WJ, Moores LK, Goodwin G, et al. An engraftment syndrome in autol-ogous stem cell transplantation related to mononuclear cell dose. Bone Marrow Transplant 2000;25:405–9.
55. Colby C, McAfee S, Sackstein R, et al. Engraftment syndrome following non-myeloablative conditioning therapy and HLA-matched bone marrow transplan-tation for hematologic malignancy. Blood 2000;96(Suppl):520.
56. Spitzer TR. Engraftment syndrome following hematopoietic stem cell transplan-tation. Bone Marrow Transplant 2001;27:893–8.
57. Takatsuka H, Takemoto Y, Yamade S, et al. Complications after bone marrow transplantation are manifestations of systemic inflammatory response syndrome. Bone Marrow Transplant 2000;26(4):419–26.
58. Woywodt A, Haubitz M, Buchholz S, et al. Counting the cost: markers of endo-thelial damage in hematopoietic stem cell transplantation. Bone Marrow Trans-plant 2004;34:1015–23.
59. Lee YH, Lim YJ, Kim JY, et al. Pre-engraftment syndrome in hematopoietic stem cell transplantation. J Korean Med Sci 2008;23:98–103.

60. Kliegman RM, Behrman RE, Jenson HB, et al. Nelson textbook of pediatrics. 18th edition. Philadelphia: Saunders Elsevier; 2007. p. 930, 1694, 2207.

61. Cesaro S, Pillon M, Talenti E, et al. A prospective survey on incidence, risk factors and therapy of hepatic veno-occlusive disease in children after hematopoietic stem cell transplantation. Haematologica 2005;90:1396–404.

62. Horn B, Reiss U, Matthay K, et al. Veno-occlusive disease of the liver in children with solid tumors undergoing autologous hematopoietic progenitor cell transplantation: a high incidence in patients with neuroblastoma. Bone Marrow Transplant 2002;29:409–15.

63. Ruutu T, Eriksson B, Remes K, et al. Ursodeoxycholic acid for the prevention of hepatic complications in allogeneic stem cell transplantation. Blood 2002;100: 1977–83.

64. Ohashi K, Tanabe J, Watanabe R, et al. The Japanese multicenter open randomized trial of ursodeoxycholic acid prophylaxis for hepatic veno-occlusive disease after stem cell transplantation. Am J Hematol 2000;64: 32–8.

65. Park SH, Lee MH, Lee H, et al. A randomized trial of heparin plus ursodial vs heparin alone to prevent hepatic veno-occlusive disease after hematopoietic stem cell transplantation. Bone Marrow Transplant 2002;29:137–43.

66. Chopra R, Eaton JD, Grassi A, et al. Defibrotide for the treatment of hepatic veno-occlusive disease: results of the European compassionate-use study. Br J Haematol 2000;111:1122–9.

67. Richardson PG, Murakami C, Jin Z, et al. Multi-institutional use of defibrotide in 88 patients after stem cell transplantation with severe veno-occlusive disease and multisystem organ failure: response without significant toxicity in a high-risk population and factors predictive of outcome. Blood 2002; 100:4337–43.

68. Chalandon Y, Roosnek E, Mermillod B, et al. Prevention of veno-occlusive disease with defibrotide after allogeneic stem cell transplantation. Biol Blood Marrow Transplant 2004;10:347–54.

69. Anasetti C, Amos D, Beatty PG, et al. Effect of HLA compatibility on engraftment of bone marrow transplants in patients with leukemia or lymphoma. N Engl J Med 1989;320(4):197–204.

70. Davies SM, Kollman C, Anasetti C, et al. Engraftment and survival after unrelated-donor bone marrow transplantation: a report for the National Marrow Donor Program. Blood 2000;96(13):4096–102.

71. Lawler M, McCann SR, Marsh JC, et al. Serial chimerism analyses indicate that mixed haemopoietic chimerism influences the probability of graft rejection and disease recurrence following allogeneic stem cell transplantation (SCT) for severe aplastic anaemia (SAA): indication for routine assessment of chimerism post SCT for SAA. Br J Haematol 2009;144:933–45.

72. Iwasaki T. Recent advances in the treatment of graft-versus-host disease. Clin Med Res 2004;2(4):243–52.

73. Afessa B, Peters SG. Major complications following hematopoietic stem cell transplantation. Semin Respir Crit Care Med 2006;27(3):297–309.

74. Wah TM, Moss HA, Robertson RJ, et al. Pulmonary complications following bone marrow transplantation. Br J Radiol 2003;76(906):373–9.

75. Khurshid I, Anderson LC. Non-infectious pulmonary complications after bone marrow transplantation. Postgrad Med J 2002;78(919):257–62.

76. Afessa B, Peters SG. Chronic lung disease after hematopoietic stem cell transplantation. Clin Chest Med 2005;26:571–86.

77. Tuthill M, Chen F, Paston S, et al. The prevention and treatment of cytomegalovirus infection in haematopoietic stem cell transplantation. Cancer Immunol Immunother 2009;58(9):1481–8.
78. Saddadi F, Najafi I, Hakemi MS, et al. Frequency, risk factors and outcome of acute kidney injury following bone marrow transplantation at Dr Shariati Hospital in Tehran. Iran J Kidney Dis 2010;4(1):20–6.
79. Michael M, Kuehnle I, Goldstein SL. Fluid overload and acute renal failure in pediatric stem cell transplant patients. Pediatr Nephrol 2004;19:91–5.
80. Patzer L, Kentouche K, Ringelmann F, et al. Renal function following hematological stem cell transplantation in childhood. Pediatr Nephrol 2003;18: 623–35.
81. Leung AY, Yuen KY, Kwong YL, et al. Polyoma BK virus and hemorrhagic cystitis in hematopoietic stem cell transplantation: a changing paradigm. Bone Marrow Transplant 2005;36:929–37.
82. Seber A, Shu XO, Defor T, et al. Risk factors for severe hemorrhagic cystitis following BMT. Bone Marrow Transplant 1999;23:35–40.
83. Comar M, D'Agaro P, Andolina M, et al. Hemorrhagic cystitis in children undergoing bone marrow transplantation: a putative role for simian virus 40. Transplantation 2004;78(4):544–8.
84. de Padua Silva L, Patah PA, Saliba RM, et al. Hemorrhagic cystitis after allogeneic hematopoietic stem cell transplants is the complex result of BK virus infection, preparative regimen intensity and donor type. Haematologica 2010;95(7): 1183–90.
85. Leung AY, Suen CK, Lie AK, et al. Quantification of polyoma BK viruria in hemorrhagic cystitis complicating bone marrow transplantation. Blood 2001;98: 1971–8.
86. Peinemann F, de Villiers EM, Dörries K, et al. Clinical course and treatment of haemorrhagic cystitis associated with BK type of human polyomavirus in nine paediatric recipients of allogeneic bone marrow transplants. Eur J Pediatr 2000;3:182–8.
87. Bhatia S, Francisco L, Carter A, et al. Late mortality after allogeneic hematopoietic cell transplantation and functional status of long-term survivors: report from the Bone Marrow Transplant Survivor Study. Blood 2007;110:3784–92.
88. Brennan BM, Shalet SM. Endocrine late effects after bone marrow transplant. Br J Haematol 2002;118:58–66.
89. Salooja N, Szydlo RM, Socie G, et al. Pregnancy outcomes after peripheral blood or bone marrow transplantation: a retrospective survey. Lancet 2001; 358:271–6.
90. Mertens AC, Ramsay NK, Kouris S, et al. Patterns of gonadal dysfunction following bone marrow transplantation. Bone Marrow Transplant 1998;22: 345–50.
91. Brauner R, Adan L, Souberbielle JC, et al. Contribution of growth hormone deficiency to the growth failure that follows bone marrow transplantation. J Pediatr 1997;130:785–92.
92. Hovi L, Rajantie J, Perkkiö M, et al. Growth failure and growth hormone deficiency in children after bone marrow transplantation for leukemia. Bone Marrow Transplant 1990;5:183–6.
93. Higman MA, Vogelsang GB. Chronic graft versus host disease. Br J Haematol 2004;125:435–54.
94. Goerner M, Gooley T, Flowers ME, et al. Morbidity and mortality of chronic GVHD after hematopoietic stem cell transplantation from HLA-identical siblings

for patients with aplastic or refractory anemias. Biol Blood Marrow Transplant 2002;8:47–56.

95. Socié G, Stone JV, Wingard JR, et al. Long-term survival and late deaths after allogeneic bone marrow transplantation. Late Effects Working Committee of the International Bone Marrow Transplant Registry. N Engl J Med 1999;341: 14–21.

96. Collaco JM, Gower WA, Mogayzel PJ Jr. Pulmonary dysfunction in pediatric hematopoietic stem cell transplant patients: overview, diagnostic considerations, and infectious complications. Pediatr Blood Cancer 2007;49(2):117–26.

97. Eikenberry M, Bartakova H, Defor T, et al. Natural history of pulmonary complications in children after bone marrow transplantation. Biol Blood Marrow Transplant 2005;11:56–64.

98. Bhatia S, Louie AD, Bhatia R, et al. Solid cancers after bone marrow transplantation. J Clin Oncol 2001;19:464–71.

99. Socié G, Curtis RE, Deeg HJ, et al. New malignant diseases after allogeneic marrow transplantation for childhood acute leukemia. J Clin Oncol 2000;18: 348–57.

100. van den Brink MR, Porter DL, Giralt S, et al. Relapse after allogeneic hematopoietic cell therapy. Biol Blood Marrow Transplant 2010;16:S138–45.

101. Cornish JM. JACIE accreditation in paediatric haemopoietic SCT. Bone Marrow Transplant 2008;42:S82–6.

102. Bevans M, Tierney DK, Bruch C, et al. Hematopoietic stem cell transplantation nursing: a practice variation study. Oncol Nurs Forum 2009;36(6):E317–25.

103. Langton H. The child with cancer: family-centred care in practice. London: Bailliere Tindall; 2000. p. 252–4.

104. Champlin RE, Horowitz MM, van Bekkum DW, et al. Graft failure following bone marrow transplantation for severe aplastic anemia: risk factors and treatment results. Blood 1989;73(2):606–13.

105. Horan JT, Carreras J, Tarima S, et al. Risk factors affecting outcome of second HLA-matched sibling donor transplantations for graft failure in severe acquired aplastic anemia. Biol Blood Marrow Transplant 2009;15:626–31.

106. Kurtzberg J, Prasad V, Carter SL, et al. Results of the Cord Blood Transplantation Study (COBLT): clinical outcomes of unrelated donor umbilical cord blood transplantation in pediatric patients with hematologic malignancies. Blood 2008;112(10):4318–27.

Ethical Considerations in Pediatric Critical Care Research

Vicki L. Zeigler, PhD, RN

KEYWORDS

• Research • Children • Ethics • Critical care

According to Beauchamp and Childress,[1(p1)] the term ethics "is a generic term for various ways of understanding the moral life." Flew[2(p112)] posits that the term ethics "suggests a set of standards by which a particular group or community decides to regulate its behavior." Yet another definition presented by Rushton[3(p108)] is more specific and states that ethics is "The study of the process for determining the best course of action in the face of conflicting choices." A less philosophic approach to ethical issues in pediatric critical care might be what was coined "clinical ethics." According to Ahronheim, Morena, and Zuckerman,[4(p2)] clinical ethics is defined as "the systematic identification, analysis, and resolution of ethical problems associated with the care of patients." The goals of clinical ethics are to protect a particular patient's interests and rights, provide assistance for health care providers in ethical decision making, and promote relationships among those close to patients that are cooperative in nature, including their health care providers and the health care institutions in which that care is provided.[4]

Regardless of the definition, nurses, in particular pediatric critical care nurses, are faced with ethical dilemmas on a daily basis as they care for their critically ill patients and their families. These ethical issues can be especially difficult when research participation of these patients is being considered and when these patients are actively participating in research studies. Although parents or legal guardians have the authority and obligation to make decisions that are best for their children, parents and legal guardians with children in critical care units report experiencing numbness as they struggle to decide what is right for the child and what is right for the family.[5] Health care professionals must bear in mind that decisions to participate in research must be value-centered and determined on an individual (patient) basis, taking into account an individual's (the patient's and the family's) personal, cultural, and religious

The author has nothing to disclose.
College of Nursing, Texas Woman's University, PO Box 425498, Denton, TX 76204-5498, USA
E-mail address: vzeigler@twu.edu

Crit Care Nurs Clin N Am 23 (2011) 377–384
doi:10.1016/j.ccell.2011.04.005   **ccnursing.theclinics.com**
0899-5885/11/$ – see front matter © 2011 Published by Elsevier Inc.

values.[6] Nurses should remain cognizant of the benefits and burdens of a particular treatment option, along with the knowledge that decision making is more difficult when the outcome is less certain.[7]

The role of the critical care nurse in pediatric research can take many directions. First and foremost, the nurse is the child's advocate and his or her role is to "commit to protecting his or her patients and to promote heath and decision making in others."[7] A myriad of research is being conducted in the pediatric critical care environment, including behavioral studies, studies involving drugs or devices, treatment modalities, and more. The pediatric critical care nurse could have the role as principal investigator in a study, could be a member of the research team, or could be the primary means of data collection. Regardless of the role played by the critical care nurse, he or she must remain cognizant of the ethical considerations inherent in pediatric critical care research.

The following discussion includes information that centers on the ethical issues of conducting research with children. First, children as a vulnerable population is explored, followed by selected ethical principles that pertain to research, the role of the technological imperative in research, the process of informed consent, and finally, nursing considerations.

CHILDREN AS A VULNERABLE POPULATION

When neonates, infants, children, and adolescents are subjects of potential research studies, researchers must recognize that they are included in the subset of research subjects that are considered "vulnerable subject populations." Vulnerable subject populations include the following individuals who require additional protections when subjects of research: (1) pregnant women, human fetuses, neonates (found in subpart B); (2) prisoners (found in subpart C); and (3) children (found in subpart D, issued in 1983).[8] Because of their associated circumstances, these individuals are likely to be vulnerable to coercion or undue influence when it comes to making decisions regarding research participation.

According to the Code of Regulations,[8] *children* "are persons who have not attained the legal age for consent to treatments or procedures involved in the research, under the applicable law of the jurisdiction in which the research will be conducted. Generally the law considers any person under 18 years old to be a child." According to Matutina,[9] there are 6 factors that contribute to the fact that children are vulnerable: (1) risks and benefits, (2) their socioeconomic status, (3) the informed consent process, (4) monetary compensation, (5) a power imbalance, and (6) confidentiality. Other causes of vulnerability for children with respect to research include (1) their lack of legal ability to provide informed consent, (2) their lack of self determination or autonomy, and (3) their cognitive abilities are not adequately developed prompting their inability to comprehend the concept of risks and benefits for research participation.[10] All of these issues make children more vulnerable for research participation, making the role of the critical care nurse as patient advocate even more important.

ASSOCIATED ETHICAL PRINCIPLES

According to Appleyard,[11] the Code of Medical Professional Ethics can be drilled down to 7 core ethical principles: (1) autonomy, (2) beneficence, (3) nonmalfeasance [sic], (4) fidelity, (5) truthfulness, (6) confidentiality, and (7) justice. The hallmark Belmont Report (a document produced in 1974 that delineated the ethical principles underlying the protection of human subjects who participate in research) centered on 3 of these principles, namely, respect for persons or autonomy, beneficence, and justice.[12] Although all of these principles are important, several are more pertinent to critical care nurses whose patients are participants in research. The following ethical principles are discussed here: (1) autonomy, which includes respect for persons; (2) beneficence; (3) veracity, which includes fidelity and truthfulness; and (4) justice.

Autonomy is defined as the right of self-determination and implies that individuals, including children, have the right to information regarding their care, particularly if it involves research. Beauchamp and Childress[1] state that respect for autonomy is a professional obligation for the health care professional and is a right, not a duty, of patients and their families. With respect to research participation, having parents provide permission for their child's participation in a study and having the child provide assent meets the principle of autonomy.[13] In essence, autonomy means making a deliberate choice regarding a specific treatment option, including whether to participate in research or not.

If parents of children in the critical care environment are to act autonomously on behalf of their children, the nurse's role is to ensure that they are adequately informed about the research study by (1) helping parents to understand any uncertainties of the disease and treatments to make a decision that is truly in the best interests of the child; (2) allowing parents the time and effort necessary to make a treatment decision, unless the child is in imminent danger of dying; (3) arranging for the availability of other health care team members, such as social services, clergy, and other ancillary services, for ongoing discussions; and (4) remembering that to accept or reject the recommended treatment options is the parent's moral decision and is not the responsibility of the health care profession.[14] Although these actions were originally set forth for the purpose of parents making health care decisions for their child, they can certainly be applied to the research process, especially the component involving informed consent.

Beneficence is another ethical principle and is defined as the act of doing goodness or kindness; beneficence requires that the nurse act in ways to promote patients' (and families') welfare.[15,16] This principle includes providing information regarding the specific beneficial aspects of a particular research study as well as risks associated with participating in the study.[1] Special consideration is directed at the benefits and risks to ensure minimal discomfort and assure the child's well being.[13] In research studies that involve anything that would promote additional anxiety for an already stressed-out child and family, such as blood drawing and other painful or invasive procedures, the provision of the information in a factual manner would meet the criteria for beneficence.

In order for the nurse to act beneficently, the information about the study and its purpose, associated benefits, and potential risks should be reviewed with the parents and their child (if applicable), while remaining cognizant of his or her obligation to respect the parent's decision to refuse to participate in a study on behalf of the child or the child's refusal to provide assent. The nurse, in a strictly advisory capacity, must show respect to patients and their families for their right to make informed health care decisions, especially when dealing with research studies, and should continue an ongoing needs assessment of the family, particularly when questions about the study arise in the data collection phase.

Veracity in the health care environment refers to the transfer of information in a comprehensive, accurate, and objective manner, as well as the fostering of the patients' and families' understanding of the information.[1] Veracity, or truth telling, which is closely tied to autonomy, is based on respect owed to others, fidelity and promise keeping, and trust.[1] The cornerstone of the nurse-patient relationship is trust, especially in keeping with the philosophy of family-centered care. Veracity in critical care nursing can be a double-edged sword in that being a patient advocate is not without risk and is directly influenced by the culture and norms of the nurse's individual practice environment.[3]

Justice has been defined by Beauchamp and Childress[1(p226)] as "fair, equitable, and appropriate treatment in light of what is due or owed to persons." According to the Belmont report,[12] "An injustice occurs when some benefit to which a person is entitled is denied without good reason or when some burden is imposed unduly." For the principle of justice to be met, the needs of individuals who are considered vulnerable populations for research, such as children, should be addressed in order for them to benefit and equal treatment should be assured.[13] For example, all pediatric patients who meet the inclusion criteria for a study should be invited to participate, regardless of their ability to pay. This behavior supports the principle of justice.

TECHNOLOGICAL IMPERATIVE

As advances in technique and other tools to aid health care providers to improve the care of their patients have evolved over the past several decades, the onslaught of new technology has added tremendously to the improvement of patient outcomes. However, along with this phenomenal increase in the availability of technology came the urgency to use it regardless of the associated costs or ramifications. This technological imperative can be defined as the pursuit of the most advanced technology and the desire to implement it without regard to cost.[17] The availability and use of technology is especially rampant in the pediatric critical care environment. According to Pohlman,[18] in a study conducted to examine the relationship of the technological imperative and the nurse-patient relationship, the notion of the technological imperative goes beyond the machinery; it is in fact a form of a technological self-understanding that transcends science, history, philosophy, and society in which individuals who come into contact with it are unconsciously unaware of its influence.[18] There is no doubt that technology has improved the care and outcomes of critically ill children, but just because the technology exists in certain circumstances does not mean there should be an obligation to use it. This point is especially illustrated in palliative end-of-life care. Although the technology might be available to prolong a child's life, at some point, families have the right to refuse that technology.

DOCUMENTATION OF INFORMED CONSENT

The informed-consent process has evolved over the years from a stance where health care professionals assumed they knew what was in the best interest of the patients and did not involve patients or families in health care decisions to a stance where it now demands that patients and families be given the needed information and then be allowed to make their own decisions.[14] These decisions should be made voluntarily and free from coercion. Although the treating physician has the responsibility to provide a recommendation for care and obtain informed consent, the nurse plays a vital role in assuring that patients and parents are informed.[13]

Informed Consent

Because children are legally unable to provide consent for research participation, informed consent is generally sought from a parent or legal guardian. According to the Code of Federal Regulations,[8] a *parent* is defined as a child's biologic or adoptive parent, whereas a *guardian* is defined as an individual who is authorized under applicable state or local law to consent on behalf of a child to general medical care. *Permission* means the agreement of a parent or guardian to the participation of their child or ward in research. Because children cannot legally provide informed consent, their parents or legal guardian provide *permission*, usually documented by the signing of an informed consent document, for their child's participation. The elements of informed consent can be found in **Table 1**.

The specific role of the nurse in the process of informed consent according to Davis[19] includes (1) monitoring and coordinating the informed-consent process, (2) being the patient advocate/liaison to the child's physician, (3) explaining alternative treatments with provision of information regarding these alternatives, and (4) being a negotiator between patients and their families and physicians when there are

Table 1
Elements of informed consent

Basic Elements	Additional Elements (When Appropriate)
1. A statement that the study involves research, an explanation of the purposes of the research, and the expected duration of the subject's participation, a description of the procedures to be followed, and identification of any procedures that are experimental	1. A statement that the particular treatment or procedure may involve risks to the subject (or to the embryo or fetus, if the subject is or may become pregnant), which are currently unforeseeable
2. A description of any reasonably foreseeable risks or discomforts to the subject	2. Anticipated circumstances under which the subject's participation may be terminated by the investigator without regard to the subject's consent
3. A description of any benefits to the subject or to others that may reasonably be expected from the research	3. Any additional costs to the subject that may result from participation in the research
4. A disclosure of appropriate alternative procedures or courses of treatment, if any, that might be advantageous to the subject	4. The consequences of a subject's decision to withdraw from the research and procedures for orderly termination of participation by the subject
5. A statement describing the extent, if any, to which confidentiality of records identifying the subject will be maintained and that notes the possibility that the Food and Drug Administration may inspect the records	5. A statement that significant new findings developed during the course of the research that may relate to the subject's willingness to continue participation will be provided to the subject
6. For research involving more than minimal risk, an explanation as to whether any compensation and an explanation as to whether any medical treatments are available if injury occurs and, if so, what they consist of, or where further information may be obtained	6. The approximate number of subjects involved in the study
7. An explanation of whom to contact for answers to pertinent questions about the research and research subject's rights, and whom to contact in the event of a research-related injury to the subject	a. A statement that informed consent requirements in these regulations are not intended to preempt any applicable federal, state, or local laws that require additional information to be disclosed for informed consent to be legally effective
8. A statement that participation is voluntary, that refusal to participate will involve no penalty or loss of benefits to which the subject is otherwise entitled, and that the subject may discontinue participation at any time without penalty or loss of benefits to which the subject is otherwise entitled	b. A statement that nothing in these regulations is intended to limit the authority of a physician to provide emergency medical care to the extent the physician is permitted to do so under applicable federal, state, or local law

From: Title 45 Code of Regulations Part §46.116, United States Department of Health and Human Services.

differences of opinion. Adequate time should be given for the parent/legal guardian to consider the information and to ask questions about study participation and the study itself.

Child Assent

Although a child may not provide legal consent to participate in research, he or she can and should provide *assent* to participate. According to Code of Federal Regulations,[8] *assent* means a child's affirmative agreement to participate in research. Mere failure to object should not, absent affirmative agreement, be construed as assent.[8] Children should also be recognized for their *dissent* to participate in research, particularly when there is no direct benefit for the child.[20] According to Gibson and Twycross,[21] the assent process should involve the provision of developmentally appropriate information to the child in order for him or her to provide assent. This information should include (1) the purpose of the research, (2) potential risks associated with the research, (3) the degree of risk (including painful procedures), (4) potential benefits, (5) the procedure for participation, and (6) identification of the members of the research team. Additionally, they recommend 2 additional topics if the research is a new or alternative treatment: (1) an explanation of the standard treatment (should one not participate in the research study) and (2) possible alternatives.[21] Adequate time should be given for the child to consider the information and to ask questions about study participation and the study itself. Although the age range required for the provision of assent varies from institution to institution, a study conducted by Tait[22] concluded that children aged 11 years or older had significantly greater understanding than children younger than 11 years with respect to research participation.

NURSING CONSIDERATIONS

According to the American Nurses Association's Code of Ethics,[23] a nurse's primary commitment is to his or her patients whether patients are individuals, families, groups, or a community. Pediatric critical care nurses have the obligation to protect the human rights of the patients whose care they provide. When caring for these children and their families, critical care nurses must recognize the importance of the ethical principles associated with research participation. Along those same lines, the critical care nurse must be aware of his or her own individual ethical conflicts. In a study conducted by Gaudine and colleagues,[24(p11)] 44 nurses and 31 physicians were interviewed regarding areas in which they experienced clinical ethical conflict. One of the 9 themes identified by both the nurses and physicians was "nurse or physician values conflict with patient values or lifestyle choices." It is extremely important that the nurse's personal values not interfere with the patients' and families' rights to consider participation in a research study. The role of the nurse is to explain the process in a way that it can be understood by patients and families in order for *them* to make their own decision about participation.

The role of the nurse within the research process does not end with informed consent. The obligation to educate patients about their care is the nurse's duty and should continue once the research study has begun. An ongoing dialog with respect to the nuances of the study with patients and their parents is paramount to ensuring the protection of human research participants, especially children. It is also important for the nurse to know that regardless of consent/assent to participate initially in a research study, the voluntary nature of research provides for participants to withdraw their participation at any time.

In summary, pediatric critical care nurses are exposed to research in the critical care environment on a routine basis and should be knowledgeable about the ethical considerations inherent in this process. Protecting their vulnerable patients, these nurses are charged with ensuring that these children and their families are well informed about potential participation in research and that based on this information the child and his or her parents are able to decide what is in the child's best interest. Realizing that more is not necessarily better, nurses must recognize the pressure placed on parents by technology, allowing them to determine a course of action with their child's health care providers with respect to that child's care. Finally, critical care nurses should graciously accept the role of patient advocate and do everything possible to protect their patients.

REFERENCES

1. Beauchamp TL, Childress JF, editors. Principles of biomedical ethics. 5th edition. New York: Oxford University Press; 2001.
2. Flew A. A dictionary of philosophy. Rev. 2nd edition. New York: Gramercy Books; 1999.
3. Rushton CH. Advocacy and moral agency: a road map for navigating ethical issues in pediatric critical care. In: Curley MA, Moloney-Harmon RA, editors. Critical care nursing of infants and children. 2nd edition. Philadelphia: W.B. Saunders Company; 2001. p. 107–27.
4. Ahronheim JC, Moreno JD, Zuckerman C, editors. Ethics in clinical practice. 2nd edition. Gaithersburg (MD): Aspen; 2000.
5. Anderson B, Hall B. Parents' perception of decision making for children. J Law Med Ethics 1995;9:1–11.
6. Pierce PF. What is an ethical decision? Crit Care Nurs Clin North Am 1997;9:1–11.
7. Mahon M. Nursing involvement in treatment decisions regarding newborns with congenital anomalies. Holist Nurs Pract 1998;2(2):55–67.
8. Code of Federal Regulations. United States Department of Health and Human Services. Office for Human Research Protections. Available at: http://www.hhs.gov/ohrp/humansubjects/guidance/45cfr46.html#46.402. Accessed September 14, 2010.
9. Matutina R. Ethical issues in research with children and young people. Paediatr Nurs 2009;21(8):38–44.
10. Hirtz DG, Fitzsimmons LG. Regulatory and ethical issues in the conduct of clinical research involving children. Curr Opin Pediatr 2002;14(6):669–75.
11. Appleyard J. Risks and benefits of research on children: developing an ethical framework to meet children's needs. Clin Risk 2008;14:215–7.
12. The Belmont Report. Ethical Principles and Guidelines for the protection of human subjects of research NIH, Department of Health Education and Welfare. Office of Human Subjects Research. Available at: http://ohsr.od.nih.gov/guidelines/belmont.html#gob3. Accessed September 14, 2010.
13. Hall JM, Stevens PE, Pletsch PK. Team research using qualitative methods: investigating children's involvement in clinical research. J Fam Nurs 2001;7: 7–31.
14. Ariff JL, Groh DH. In the best interest of the child: ethical issues. In: Curley MA, Smith JB, Moloney-Harmon PA, editors. Critical care nursing of infants and children. Philadelphia: W.B. Saunders; 1996. p. 126–41.
15. Burkhardt MA, Nathaniel AK. Ethics and issues in contemporary nursing. Albany (NY): Delmar Publications; 1998.
16. Mappes TA, DeGrazia D. General introduction. In: Mappes TA, DeGrazia D, editors. Biomedical ethics. 5th edition. New York: McGraw-Hill; 2001. p. 1–55.

17. Herhold S. The technological imperative in United States healthcare. 2007. Available at: www.cs.virginia.edu/~acw/REU/Herhold.ppt. Accessed September 20, 2010.
18. Pohlman S. Fathering premature infants and the technological imperative of the neonatal intensive care unit. ANS Adv Nurs Sci 2009;32(3):E1–16.
19. Davis AJ. Clinical nurses' ethical decision making in situations of informed consent. ANS Adv Nurs Sci 1989;12:63–9.
20. Schwenzer KJ. Protecting vulnerable subjects in clinical research: children, pregnant women, prisoners, and employees. Respir Care 2008;53(10):1342–9.
21. Gibson F, Twycross A. Children's participation in research. A position statement on behalf of the Royal College of Nursing's Research in Child Health (RiCH) group and Children's and Young People's Rights and Ethics Group. Paediatr Nurs 2007; 19(4):14–7.
22. Tait AR, Voepel-Lewis T, Shobha M. Do they understand (part II). Assent of children participating in clinical anesthesia and surgery research. Respir Care 2003; 98(6):609–14.
23. American Nurses Association. Code of ethics for nurses with interpretive statements. 2010. Available at: http://www.nursingworld.org/MainMenuCategories/EthicsStandards/CodeofEthicsforNurses/Code-of-Ethics.aspx. Accessed October 15, 2010.
24. Gaudine A, LeFort SM, Lamb M, et al. Clinical ethical conflicts of nurses and physicians. Nurs Ethics 2011;18(1):9–19.

Index

Note: Page numbers of article titles are in **boldface** type.

Crit Care Nurs Clin N Am 23 (2011) 385–392
doi:10.1016/S0899-5885(11)00020-7
0899-5885/11/$ – see front matter © 2011 Elsevier Inc. All rights reserved.

ccnursing.theclinics.com

Moving?

Make sure your subscription moves with you!

To notify us of your new address, find your **Clinics Account Number** (located on your mailing label above your name), and contact customer service at:

Email: journalscustomerservice-usa@elsevier.com

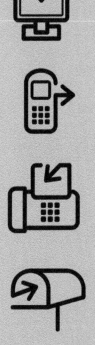

800-654-2452 (subscribers in the U.S. & Canada)
314-447-8871 (subscribers outside of the U.S. & Canada)

Fax number: 314-447-8029

Elsevier Health Sciences Division
Subscription Customer Service
3251 Riverport Lane
Maryland Heights, MO 63043

*To ensure uninterrupted delivery of your subscription, please notify us at least 4 weeks in advance of move.

ELSEVIER

Printed and bound by CPI Group (UK) Ltd, Croydon, CR0 4YY

03/10/2024

01040448-0020